GRAY MATTER

WHY YOU MUST SAFEGUARD YOUR AGED RELATIVES SO THAT THEY CAN LIVE HAPPILY AFTER RETIREMENT FOR 30 YEARS OR MORE

Edited by

Isaac Ato Mensah

and

Florence Afful

Publishers

www.writersghana.com

DEDICATION

To our parents and all aged persons

ACKNOWLEDGEMENTS

Thank you Kairos Emmanuel for offering the assistance that made sharing of documents and collaborating on this book project from different locations at the same time possible. Thank you Augustine Ato Kakraba for proofreading the initial and final manuscript. Florence Afful, the co-editor, played a unique "safeguarding" role of asking the critical questions and playing the skeptical vanguard role that kept the ship on an even keel. We appreciate our indefatigable mentees at www.writersghana.com who play diverse roles in getting our research and writing in shape. Thank you Dr NAB Andrews, world renowned neurosurgeon, for the mentorship. And of course, we are very grateful to Mr Saed Nyarko who answers all our IT questions.

PREFACE

The proverb "a rolling stone gathers no moss" could be interpreted in at least two ways. Firstly, the original perspective - call it British - is that permanency of tenure of employment helps one to gain experience/expertise and become more grounded with a wealth of knowledge in a particular subject matter. The other perspective is that the inefficiencies and disadvantages that you accrue by staying at one place become, as it were, a moss - algae, Spirogyra, warts and all - which must be avoided by rolling on from one job experience to the other.

The four authors thus sharing their experiences/expertise in this book are using triangulation - both literally and symbolically - to corroborate their argument. In the literal sense, one set of evidence from the respective authors' experiences/expertise and the latest literature, are being used to corroborate the other. In the symbolic sense, the four authors share previous and current experiences/expertise from three continents - North America (USA), Europe (the UK) and Africa (Ghana). The book is further made rich with empirical evidence from journal articles.

One key objective of this book is to show that the experiences/observations of the authors are consistent with the empirical evidence from the latest literature and best practice guidelines. Hence the authors have sufficient credible experience/expertise for teaching and offering guidance on safeguarding the aged. What is more, the proposals made in this book - our gray matter - for safeguarding in a nursing care home as well as assisted living can be implemented in any district assembly or local council or local government that seeks to implement a serious population health program. In other words, the book is more about why safeguarding is needed and less about how to do safeguarding.

But more to the point, our overarching objective is to convincingly drive home the point that safeguarding the aged is for everyone. The book offers important perspectives, and hence provokes a healthy public discourse about safeguarding the aged everywhere as a population health imperative.

Isaac Ato Mensah

11 July, 2023

Accra

TABLE OF CONTENTS

1

INTRODUCTION

Isaac Ato Mensah

Florence Afful

People are getting older everywhere on Earth. Of course it is because they are living longer, isn't it? (Roser et al., 2019; Rural Health Information Hub, n.d.). This is a happy problem. The challenge? Assistance with daily living. Living with dementia and other comorbidities. You're happy and joyous that granny and gramps are alive. Good. You're perhaps planning their birthday party. The implication of your happiness is that it presents a daily problem - a duty of care, the need to reduce pain - for some people. These people are healthcare managers, carers/caregivers, professional Nurses, Medical Doctors, a multidisciplinary team of healthcare workers in every land and clime (American Hospital Association, 2014). Of course they do get paid. But, they need you to make their client - no, your relative - happy, happier, happiest, all the days of their lives. The aim of this book, therefore, is to conceptualize and present safeguarding the aged as a population health issue of concern, to wit, a gray matter. This gray matter has reached crisis levels. Now here's the thing: you can help. We're all called to heal, aren't we? In this book we expose the problem and its implications. We then present some solutions. Next, we invite you to also add yours. Why? Because ideas are universal, simpliciter! Therefore, no matter your status in the scheme of things: a private individual, family leadership, WhatsApp and other social media groups enforcer, community leader, street captain, local government leader - you can fashion out your own unique innovative solution to address the challenge. This is for at least one reason: all human beings - you and us - desire to grow old while pursuing happiness (Taylor, 2018). Indeed as the ancient philosopher Plato pointed out in The Republic, "a life committed to knowledge and virtue will result in happiness" (Johnson, 2022, para. 37). That is why we invite you to join us in pursuing this gray matter that brings happiness to mankind. We all wish to become seniors in our families and communities, don't we? During such periods in our lives, we could become more vulnerable.

Today, value-based care has been established as the way to go. And assisted living is part of that paradigm shift (Neufeld, 2017). To make our argument convincing, we analyze data from King County in Washington State, USA, to demonstrate a high income country context. We then analyze similar data for Western North Region, Upper West Region, Upper East Region, and Savannah Region in Ghana. This enables us to demonstrate the context of a Low and Middle Income Country. Low and Middle Income countries (LMICs) are "a diverse group by size, population, and income level…..defined as lower middle-income economies - those with a GNI [gross national income] per capita between [US]$1,036 and [US]$4,045; and upper middle-income economies - those with a GNI per capita between [US]$4,046 and [US]$12,535. Middle income countries are home to 75% of the world's population and 62% of the world's poor" (The World Bank, 2022, para. 1).

We then propose five assisted living programs. The first is for King County in Washington State, USA. Two of the four authors of this book live in Washington State, but not necessarily in King County. The second proposed assisted living program is for the Western North Region. The third is for the Upper West Region. The fourth, for the Upper East Region and the fifth for the Savannah Region. All four authors hail from Ghana, but none of us hail from the aforementioned selected regions. The four regions in Ghana and King County in Washington State, U.S.A., were all selected based on their demographics. These demographics reveal peculiar population health needs/challenges that justify our choices.

We also look at some data which explain the need for safeguarding the aged within an assisted living program. Later in this book, we explain what is unique about our proposed King County Assisted Living Program (KCALP). We also hereby make a similar proposal for four of the most rural regions of Ghana based on the same concept as the KCALP. Our model is only a guide based on facts, evidence and reason. Any person, therefore, armed with a similar set of facts as ours should select any district in their country and make a similar case for a local government sponsored assisted living program. We have also shared with you caregiving under an assisted living program at home, in a residential care home, or in a nursing care home. This book, thus discusses both the raison d'etre and the know-how - das know-how, Fachwissen - of caregiving.

Even though we discuss practical experiences/expertise from the U.S., U.K., and Ghana throughout this book, we mostly use data for the United States and Ghana, so that you, the reader, may have the clearest global picture. Those two countries, that is, the U.S. and Ghana, do not have universal health insurance. Ghana is a quintessential Low and Middle Income Country which also represents the Global South. The United States is one of the three Organization for Economic Cooperation and Development (OECD) Member countries which do not have universal health insurance (OECD, 2015). The other two OECD Member countries without universal health insurance, namely, Greece and Poland, are not listed in the Top 20 richest countries in the world in 2022. But the U.S. makes that list (Kovacevic, 2022). At the same time the U.S. represents the Global North. Safeguarding the aged through assisted living as per this gray matter is an important wealth distribution concept, hence there is no reason why the wealthiest nation on Earth should not adopt it. We hope that by the purposive sampling of Ghana, the U.K., and the U.S., our gray matter will be adopted/adapted by much of the world.

There are at least 46 million Americans who are above 65 years (Rural Health Information Hub, n.d.). Do you already foresee more undocumented migrants in America and other parts of the high income countries seeking Carer/Caregiver jobs? Beyond the U.S. data, life expectancy has generally increased globally over the last 100 years. This is primarily due to improvement in medicine, diet, vaccines and social amenities, among other factors (Roser et al., 2019). This means that for people who have suffered historical trauma, managing themselves alone at home while living longer with comorbidities is an additional burden that requires some intervention (Harvard University, n.d.; Harris, 2014; alchemicalmedia, 2013). Issues of historical trauma are known to be indicative of lifetime diseases including chronic diseases which develop in later life (Harvard University, n.d.; Harris, 2014; alchemicalmedia, 2013). You will read about historical trauma extensively in this book.

Income inequality is also a problem that exacerbates the problem of seniors who have suffered historical trauma. The picture is equally stark when one looks at the data for severe housing problems. At least 405000 people in King County have severe housing problems. This gray matter/innovative solution more directly addresses the domain of risk prevention and reduction, especially the risk of falling which oldies suffer a lot. When people who need assisted living are injured at home, the health and financial ramifications may become a logistical nightmare including relatives losing working hours in order to give more attention to the injured elderly. This is all preventable - 75% of the time (Alvarez et al., 2015). But we need taxpayers' money to better promote assisted living. Even in the UK, with some of the best practice safeguarding systems for the aged, the plight of illegal/undocumented immigrants when they reach age 60 is a gray matter that cannot be swept under the carpet.

Indigenous peoples, especially people who have suffered historical trauma, generally have been let down by society. This is the time for restoration; this is the time to give back that which was lost. One day we shall all become old, hopefully, and will need support with assisted living either in our own homes, preferably, or in a nursing care home. Assisted Living is an essential part of value-based care. Any local government authority which adopts the prospectus freely given in this book will no doubt show commitment to addressing the problems created by historical trauma, especially trauma suffered by indigenous peoples.

Boland et al. (2017) found no differences in health outcomes between rehabilitation at home versus conventional rehabilitation services. However, assisted living will be cheaper for the King County Government and the aforementioned four Ghanaian regions to implement since the clients/subscribers will live in their own homes. Indeed, it will be cheaper in the end, for every nation on earth without effective old age care programs to adopt this gray matter. This gray matter is a sustainable innovation strategy under the Sustainable Development Goals (SDGs) (Danish Institute for Human Rights, n.d.; Christensen et al., 2015). Item 1.3 of the SDGs advocates that by 2030, countries should implement nationally appropriate social protection systems that cover the vulnerable (Danish Institute for Human Rights, n.d.). We are hereby and herewith leading evidence through these pages to demonstrate that this gray matter is in tandem with that worthy global agenda.

Finally, since at least 1958, through the machinations of the airline industry and the Federal Aviation Authority of the United States, age 60 has come to be accepted worldwide as the conventional age of retirement (Francis, 2005). Since the 2008 global financial crisis, however, there have been attempts at delaying the retirement age to 64, 65, 67 years, et cetera, in many jurisdictions. The reason is not difficult to fathom: pension funds are going broke. Pension funds across the world are struggling to live up to their respective promises mainly because pensioners are living longer; way beyond when they are expected to die, to put it bluntly. Ironically, back in 1958, airline pilots - and workers generally for that matter - wanted to keep working until they were physically and or mentally unfit to continue working (Francis, 2005). In many jurisdictions, the respective retirement ages have not changed. In other places, there are protests against increasing the retirement age. Our considered view is that since many living pensioners were retired at age 60, we should keep this gray matter reference point as age 60 when seniors are psychologically attuned to going on retirement.

2

WHY SAFEGUARDING THE AGED?

Isaac Ato Mensah

Florence Afful

SAFEGUARDING DEFINED

We define Safeguarding as protecting the aged, vulnerable children and people with learning disabilities from their exploiters, neighbors, family and even those that give them care/support in their daily living. Thus safeguarding is a system whereby the above-mentioned persons are protected. It is everybody's responsibility to protect the vulnerable and elderly especially in a care setting. Hence we can say that safeguarding is a process whereby vulnerable people are protected from all sorts of harm. The harm could be physical, it could be emotional, it could be sexual, and/or it could be financial. So long as vulnerable persons are protected from any exploitation and even self harm, we are safeguarding them.

It is hereby proposed that the King County government should pay for assisted living services for indigenous people. Ditto for the district assemblies under the Western North Region, Savannah Region, Upper West Region and Upper East Region of Ghana. In addition, to avoid discrimination, all aged persons who will need assisted living should equally be supported by the King County Government. In the case of Ghana, the respective district assemblies should use their health units to coordinate/lead this task.

The metrics for the Second Curve of Health Care enables hospital leaders to evaluate current position and progress along the continuum toward meeting second-curve metrics, namely providing value-based care (Health Research and

Educational Trust, 2013). Assisted living for the aged who are needy will, therefore, help address value-based care (Neufeld, 2017).

The fact that health systems around the world are seeing the need to offer more home-based care, person centered care, and whole-person care in some cases, show a shift from volume-based care to value-based care. According to the United Nations, the number of people who are 65 years or older grew larger than children under the age of five in 2018 (United Nations, n.d). This trend will continue such that by 2050, that is, 27 years from today, within a generation, out of every six persons on Earth one will be older than 65 years old (United Nations, n.d.). By analogy, the situation will be like the way some people used to say that out of every six persons on earth, one is Indian, or one is Chinese. For many people in Low and Middle Income Countries, the dependency ratio will increase. And these are the countries who have very low disposable incomes such that they cannot afford assisted living services.

What is more, issues of historical trauma are known to be indicative of lifetime diseases including chronic diseases which develop in later life (Harris, 2014). Finally, access to exercise opportunities - 98% for King County; 87% for Washington State; and 91% for the top U.S. performers - offers a glimmer of hope that with careful strategic planning involving community leaders and community people some health parameters can be improved (County Health Rankings and Roadmap, n.d.). All such data are publicly available and more will be delved into so that a clear solution based on data could be obtained. For sure, the plight of indigenous peoples around the world is evidence that historical trauma has devastating consequences. Many of these people may need assisted living.

THE DOMAIN OF SAFEGUARDING

Safeguarding is a very broad concept. In this book we have chosen to focus on safeguarding the aged. Even so, we have focused more on the why of safeguarding and less on the how of safeguarding for several reasons. First, there are many credible textbooks out there that discuss various aspects of safeguarding. Second, there are various laws and regulations in various jurisdictions that address safeguarding of the aged. Often, it is preferred that if you are a carer, or nurse in the UK, for example, you do not read American textbooks on safeguarding, otherwise you may end up with a poor understanding of the relevant legislation and guidelines for action. The reverse is true. Ditto for safeguarding in say Germany, Finland, Russia, China, or Japan. Third, there are various websites that freely offer important lessons on safeguarding. Those learning resources discuss safeguarding topics such as duty of care, infection prevention, cyber fraud, how to prevent abuse, and financial abuse, to name but a few. Our book simply places all of that in context and makes a strong case that safeguarding the aged is an existential population health crisis - or gray matter - that must immediately arrest the attention of public health/population health officials. When such officials - and you the reader - understand why this matter must be the concern of all, then humankind can collaborate on various levels and across multi-sectoral lines to address the subject matter.

Please find below a list of relevant institutions and their websites that are useful learning resources about safeguarding:

1) National Institute for Care and Health Excellence (UK),
   https://www.nice.org.uk/
2) Grey Matter Learning (UK).
   https://greymatterlearning.co.uk/course/safeguarding-for-managers-and-safeg
   uarding-leads/#course_intro
3) The Carents Room (UK). https://carents.co.uk/about/
4) SAFEcic https://www.safecic.co.uk/home/about-us#background
5) ageUK.
   https://www.ageuk.org.uk/globalassets/age-ni/documents/factsheets/fs78_safe
   guarding_older_people_from_abuse_fcs.pdf

6) Social Care Institute for Excellence
https://www.scie.org.uk/person-centred-care/older-people-care-homes/safety

7) NHS England North Designated Professionals for Safeguarding Adults.
https://www.england.nhs.uk/wp-content/uploads/2017/02/adult-pocket-guide.pdf

8) Government Accountability Office (US).
https://www.gao.gov/products/gao-19-599

9) Administration on Aging (US). https://acl.gov/about-acl/administration-aging

10) Consumer Financial Protection Bureau (US).
https://www.consumerfinance.gov/consumer-tools/educator-tools/resources-for-older-adults/protecting-against-fraud/#resources-for-consumers

11) The United States Department of Justice.
https://www.justice.gov/elderjustice/prosecutors/statutes

12) Centers for Disease Control and Prevention (US).
https://www.cdc.gov/violenceprevention/elderabuse/fastfact.html

13) Humanitas (Germany).
https://www.humanitas-pflegeservice.de/11-0-Homecare+Eldercare.html

14) European Parliament (EU/Germany).
https://www.europarl.europa.eu/RegData/etudes/STUD/2021/662940/IPOL_STU(2021)662940(ANN03)_EN.pdf

15) Attorney-General's Department (Australia).
https://www.ag.gov.au/rights-and-protections/protecting-rights-older-australians

16) Help Age (Ghana and West Africa).
https://www.helpage.org/global-network/africa/west-africa/

17) Western Cape Government (South Africa).
https://www.westerncape.gov.za/assets/departments/social-development/south_african_policy_for_older_persons_2005.pdf

BIDDING BED SORES TO HEAL FAST

Florence Afful

Since this book is for everyone, we have incorporated topics that should serve as self help guides for non-professionals who may offer caregiving at home. Or even in a residential care home/nursing care home as they visit their relatives. It is also in your interest to know exactly what the Carers/Nurses are expected to do. We all may through that become more empathetic and supportive. Or armed with this knowledge, successfully report abuse. One of the burning issues in safeguarding the aged is managing bedsores. Those who are already handling assisted living at home, in a residential care home, or in a nursing care home will be familiar with this huge problem which borders on neglect of the resident. In this chapter, we offer some best practice guidelines in the hope that caregivers and relatives alike may find support from this literature as a basis for asking critical questions when things go wrong.

Bedridden residents with restricted mobility are those that are prone to developing pressure sores. With pressure sores, the management is in a few ways. One sure way is ensuring that they do not stay in their urine. This is done by changing their clothing including pads promptly. You do not let them stay in the urine and the poop. This is because chemicals in the urine and the poop enter the skin. For the elderly, their circulation is poor because they are not moving about easily so they are prone to developing sores. Hence, make sure they are changed regularly. Changing such persons regularly is part of incontinent care which is taught to nursing students. Therefore, as a relative, you may politely ask the Nurse or Caregiver why they are not changing your elderly relative regularly. And we bet the discussion will be interesting. You should not leave the residents or elderly to stay in their urine or poop for so long; that is not best practice.

Then we come to Positioning. This refers to turning the resident hourly, or two-hourly, or three-hourly depending on the need of the resident or the severity of the sores that have already developed. You also do repositioning as a preventive measure for those that are bedridden and unable to move or turn themselves to relieve the pressure on the part of the body against the bed. For such persons there is pressure and friction that is created between the body and the bed. So if the person is bed-bound or chair-bound and is unable to move, especially stroke sufferers, they need regular turning. On an hourly or two-hourly basis, you should turn them depending on the severity of the case. Nutrition also plays an essential part in pressure sore management (Hardman et al., 2015). Please make sure that residents get their high protein diet and fluids to improve the pressure situation. There are pressure relieving mattresses/air mattresses and pressure cushions that are available to prevent and treat persons with pressure sores or who are prone to developing pressure sores. The pressure relieving mattresses/air mattresses are used when the client is in bed. Its purpose is to relieve the pressure on the skin. The air inside is inflated in alternating fashion so that the pressure on the skin from the part of the body lying on the bed is reduced. In managing pressure sores effectively, you have to manage the client's hydration and their diet carefully. Please ensure to give them a balanced diet when they have developed a sore. You have to be dressing the sore. You need to involve the tissue viability nurse who is a specialist in managing ulcers.

4

A FALL IS A FALL

Florence Afful

Just as the previous chapter on managing bedsores, the phenomenon of aged persons falling down is an important gray matter. Falls occur at home, in a residential care home, or in a nursing care home. Indeed a fall can occur anywhere. These guidelines should help offer some important teaching points to everyone who is needed to support direct healthcare workers in safeguarding residents.

Falls are caused due to so many factors, but we may classify them into two broad categories: medical and physical causes. The medical reasons could be due to medication side effects. If the causes are medication side effects, then there could be a medication review so that the medication is given at night when the resident is going to bed. However, some residents may be on medication for day and night. If that's the case then you need regular monitoring to make sure the resident doesn't fall. Now let's discuss the details of how to prevent falls.

Falls can happen to anyone. In the case of a resident with unsteady gait or a person living with dementia whose mobility is poor yet they still think they can walk, managing falls is an important gray matter. They are unsteady, but due to dementia they think they can walk so they just get up and then they end up falling down.

Persons with walking aids such as Zimmer frames and wheelchairs also end up falling often. Even those lying in bed sometimes need bed rails pulled up or down in order to prevent falls. There are usually bumpers or cushion covers on the rails to prevent them from falling down the bed. The other one is if residents are not wearing the right clothing such as well-fitting shoes, they could end up falling down. So then what do we do?

Firstly, we need to make sure the aged person's surroundings are always well lit and cluster-free. If a resident is prone to falling down from the bed, the measure we put in place is that when the resident is first admitted, or you take over the home care job, you have to assess and determine whether the person has anxieties and moves about in bed. If the resident is like that then putting in place a bed rail (cotside) is risky because the person can put the legs in between the bed rail (cotside) and get bruises, or they can choke and die.

There are at least two ways out of this situation. First, if the person can lie down calmly, then you provide a low profile bed. A low profile bed is way, way down; lowered so low such that when the person falls down from the bed onto the floor, there should not be that much injury. Also we provide a crash mattress and or sensor mattress, depending on the need. If the person has the tendency of getting up and trying to walk and you know they are at risk, you place the crash mattress on the floor plus the sensor mattress on top of it. The sensor mattress is just connected to the culvert so immediately the person gets up and puts the legs down the sensor mattress will ring. The crash mattress is just like the normal mattress you sleep on. Just place it on the floor in front of the bed, depending on the position of the bed.

Sometimes we place the mattresses on both sides of the bed, but if the bed is against a wall, then of course you place the crash mattress on only one side on the floor. If somebody is falling because of clothing, obviously you have to make sure the person gets the right clothing. The right clothing includes the right shoe size, the right pants (trousers), or joggers to wear. When it comes to moving and handling, residents can fall if you do not check the equipment promptly before using it to move them. Therefore, make sure you check your equipment promptly, ensuring they are in working order before you go and move anyone in them. If somebody falls, but there is no injury, please observe first and satisfy yourself that the person did not get any injuries. Then of course two persons should help move the resident depending on their mobility plan.

If the resident needs hoisting, to be hoisted up, two persons should hold the person to stand if the resident can stand. If the person is injured then you do not move the person. Depending on the injury, you may leave the person there on the floor and ensure they are comfortable. Protect the person from any dangers on the floor and then you call the ambulance depending on the telephone number used in your jurisdiction. But if there is no injury, then of course assist the person from off the floor and do your neurological observations for 48 hours. Every 30 minutes, and then one hour and then two hours for 48 hours. If you can get access to inform the residents General Practitioner, or Specialist please do so. Then fill your incident forms. For sure you have to inform the relatives about it. If you do not inform the relatives and fill out the incident forms, if something is noticed, it becomes a safeguarding issue of abuse against you, the caregiver who had a duty of care at the time. There are some types of medication that make a patient drowsy and thus prone to falls. In such cases you have to make sure the Medical Doctors review the medications the residents are taking.

What do you do when a patient is agitated and jumping in and out of bed?

With those ones you cannot use bed rails. If you do, they will try to jump out of bed or put their legs through the spaces in them. People have died through such unfortunate situations. The best approach is to use a low profile bed so that when the person falls they may not be injured. Then you put crash mattresses at the exposed sides. Of course, again, if the bed is beside a wall, then only one crash mattress is placed at one side. Straps may also be used for residents sitting in a wheelchair; you need to be authorized by the relevant regulatory authority before you use them on a resident. Otherwise it could be misconstrued as restricting the freedoms of such residents who otherwise need them. The best practice approach (as exemplified by the UK) is to apply for Denial of Liberty (DOL) from the relevant authorities.

Sometimes some residents will come out of bed and try to walk or crawl. Since they are unstable, this could be dangerous as they may fall down and get themselves injured. Here is where the sensor mattress comes in (Sangeetha et al., 2022). The sensor mattress is put on the crash mattress which is lying on the floor on one or both sides of the bed depending on location. With the slightest pressure on it, the sensor mattress rings. Everybody will hear the sound so that when you hear it you know that the resident has come out of bed. You have to go and check what the situation is. The advantage here is that some residents do not know how to use the call bell which is why they come out of bed without calling for assistance. The sensor mattress is connected to the call bell so when it rings and everybody including the staff hear it, they have to look on their computer screen to know which room the sound is coming from. When staff are on duty, they need to know which rooms have been supplied with sensor mattresses. When you are also going to give care at the bedside and you step on the crash mattress it rings. Thus it is easy to identify a crash mattress. All told, persons with mobility problems need sensor mattresses around them so that immediately they move, then you go and see what the situation is.

SUMMARY

On falls, you have to review the medication and see if it is causing falls. Then refer the resident to the fall clinic. Next, review the resident's mobility care plan if need be. This means you have to review your processes. Is it clothing? Shoes? Is it the arrangements in the room? You can do all the right things and the resident may still fall. A fall is a fall; be vigilant.

Back to the Zimmer frame. Please do not go out there and just buy any Zimmer frame. Zimmer frames must be assessed for their weight and height. Ditto for the other walking aids. These assessments should be done by the physiotherapist. This way the right ones will be selected based on what is good for the mobility of the resident.

Back also to the hoisting. Please make sure the machine is in good working condition. No one should fall out of a hoisting machine. That would be terrible, wouldn't it?

Back yet again to the agitated patient. Is the person someone who rolls over when sleeping? Is it someone whose mobility is limited so they just lie still? Or is it someone who doesn't make any moves that will suggest to you that they may fall? The usual approach is to provide a low profile bed.

You should check their diet also. Are they hungry? Are they confused? Do they have urinary tract infections (UTIs)? Some of these elderly people do not drink much fluids. Some carers also do not have the patience to feed the residents well and give them fluids. When this happens such deprived residents may develop recurrent UTIs. This makes them agitated and confused. Hence you have to check and make sure that there is no underlying medical condition that makes the residents confused, thereby falling. Make sure the resident has a balanced diet. Sometimes the pads are wet. Other times the pads may not have been changed by the carers. Sometimes the residents cannot talk so they try to get up. That results in falls. Sometimes the residents want to go to the toilet. If they are not able to communicate this, they may try to get up. Also, if the residents are otherwise feeling uncomfortable, they may try to get up.

WHEN TO CALL THE TELEMEDICINE TEAM

Isaac Ato Mensah

Florence Afful

The Covid-19 pandemic and its aftermath have highlighted the relevance of telemedicine even in environments without established protocols for telemedicine. In nursing care homes, there may not be many medical doctors and specialists assigned for all residents. One, therefore, has to work with the telemedicine team whose duty it is to recommend that the patient should be taken to hospital (Giannulli, 2014).

The recent ambulance booking delays in the UK which forced many people to take their relatives to hospital by themselves "during a lengthy emergency", has underscored the growing importance of telemedicine (Sharma, 2023, para. 1). "One in three people said that they have had to drive or even take public transport to provide emergency care to their loved ones because of delays in ambulance response, revealed a poll by the Liberal Democrats" (Sharma, 2023, para. 2).

How is this story different from a similar narrative you may have read or heard about from say rural Bangladesh, Bolivia, Brazil, Ceylon, Chile, Indonesia, Kenya, Nigeria, Uganda, Zambia and/or Zimbabwe? Maybe the addition to the narrative from the low and middle income countries is that the patient was conveyed to a health center on a tricycle, taxi, Okada (commercial passenger motorbike rides in Nigeria; also now called Okada in Ghana), or a passenger bus (christened Trotro in Ghana and Danfo in Nigeria).

The situation is no doubt worse in Low and Middle Income Countries (LMICs) where there are inadequate ambulance services. Therefore, the work of the nurse and the telemedicine team are very crucial and complementary. Needless to say there are cost implications for making a judgment call that a resident should be taken to hospital. And all of that largely depends on the Nurse. If you have good records and have managed your residents well, your judgment call will be vindicated. Otherwise, the third-party of even resident financiers will hold you to account. This has implications for your license renewal with the Nurses and Midwives Council (NMC) of the UK, or their equivalent organization in whatever jurisdiction you find yourself in.

So let us learn and refresh our minds on what to do with the concerns of residents, colleagues, relations, the ambulance team, and the telemedicine team before making a final decision. Nurses already know what to do when transferring a resident to a hospital and back to the care facility. One cannot bear mentioning enough that documentation is key to success. It will help to troubleshoot the system and retrace your steps should something go wrong. The particular protocol you will follow depends on your care facility. However, there surely are some common sense rules that should apply to all. It is not always that the telemedicine team recommends hospital transfer. They sometimes make Medical Doctors assess the patient via a video call after which treatment is started. Finally, please always remember that calling the telemedicine team has financial cost implications.

ACTIVE LISTENING

Isaac Ato Mensah

Florence Afful

The objective of this chapter is to assist you in improving your active listening skills. We have prepared a self appraisal checklist to assess active listening. It is our fervent hope that you will use the appraisal checklist to get positive feedback from patients, patients' relatives and colleagues. Such feedback will indicate that you, the reader, have improved in your listening and interaction abilities.

In order to listen actively, one must pay attention to the speaker's aim, feeling, and content. The individual who is actively listening expresses attention by asking questions and by giving nonverbal and visual indicators that the speaker is making critical points.

Ineffective communication is one of the major contributors to medical mistakes and accidental injury to patients. Listening is a crucial component of this skill called active listening. And yes, active listening is a skill because it can be taught and learnt. The main objective of this chapter is thus pretty clear: to teach, learn and promote active listening.

In rushed conversations between two persons, active listening rarely happens (Jahromi et al., 2016). This skill involves both verbal and nonverbal components, and in order to be a good active listener, various factors should be taken into account. Such factors include appropriate body language and "posture showing involvement, facial expressions, eye contact", and expressing interest in the speaker's words (Jahromi et al., 2016, para. 5). In addition, minimal verbal encouragement, attentive silence, reflecting back feelings and content, and intellectually summarizing the speaker's words and their purpose should also be done (Jahromi et al., 2016). There are three main aspects of active listening that we may use as parameters to judge our listening acumen: "listening attitude, listening skill, and conversation opportunity" (Jahromi et al., 2016, para. 5).

THE FLORENCE-ATO-MENSAH ACTIVE LISTENING SCORE

We hereby use the parameters suggested by Jahromi et al. (2016) based on their research, to develop The Florence-Ato-Mensah Active Listening Score. It is a checklist of 15 questions.

Were there interruptions from staff/clients? - Yes [0] No [1]

Did you yawn during the listening process?

Yes [0] No [1]

Did you snap/get upset?

Yes [0] No [1]

Did you promptly apologize after an interruption?

Yes [0] No [1]

Did you look at /touch your watch, phone or other device as if to suggest that the person was wasting your time?

Yes [0] No [1]

How often did you look at /touch your watch, phone or other device within 30 minutes?

Often [0] hardly [1]

How often did you interrupt to conclude on what the speaker was saying?

Often [0] hardly [1]

Did you take notes according to the prescribed nursing format?

Yes [1] No [0]

Did you summarize the points being raised orally for confirmation by the speaker?

Yes [1] No [0]

Will you be able to prepare the resident's care plan from the information obtained?

Yes [1] No [0]

Will you be able to complete all the regulatory agencies' required documentation from the information obtained?

Yes [1] No [0]

Have you confirmed that the client has an active contact line/address such that when they leave you can get in touch and retrieve the same information if you lose what you have documented?

Yes [1] No [0]

Did you maintain eye contact?

Yes [1] No [0]

Did the interviewee/speaker express appreciation for your effort?

Yes [1] No [0]

Were you able to complete and submit all your reports before handing over duty such that the one taking over can continue caregiving?

Yes [1] No [0]

Total Florence-Ato-Mensah Active Listening Score: Yes [15] No [0]

Since we should all aim for the highest ideals, all 15 questions are crucially important. Therefore, if you scored less than 15, then you have not mastered active listening. Anything less than 15 means you need self improvement. You may never know the one mistake that could mess up your entire effort. We all need to improve don't we? Is it possible that you may do well in some environments and less than optimal in other contexts? Please try this scale across various situations and see how you perform in various places and over time. Is there anything else you may want to add to this active listening checklist?

CAN ALL STAFF BE TRAINED TO GIVE THE SAME MINIMUM STANDARD OF CARE?

Isaac Ato Mensah

Barbara Vanessa Sabbi

We take the liberty to assume that every employer will hire staff who can exercise sound judgment when duty calls. To address the debate about whether some persons are more affable than others and/or whether affability can be learnt, we refer to the literature. The conclusion is yours to do. But for sure, there are some minimum acceptable standards for the caregiving vocation. And yes, caregiving is a vocation. If you do not accept that, then we suggest you go look for another job. Please remember that any razzmatazz/Jombolijo attitude you display could result in negligence and neglect. And you know the consequences, right? Prepare for a protracted litigation. Your employer/facility/supervisors won't be spared either.

Turkheimer has observed that in nonhuman animals, the nature–nurture debate can be more easily resolved through experiments whereas in humans, there are ethical inhibitions (n.d.). At the same time, humankind's ability to play basketball or the violin excellently, for example, could be due to some diet which may have benefitted them with time. Much of what we know about nature vs nurture comes from studying animals, not people. Adoption studies and observing twins are very ethical ways by which to study human behavior (Turkheimer, n.d.). With adopted children, we can tell if the environment has an effect on their behavior or that the children will manifest what is in their genes (Turkheimer, n.d.). Twins and adopted children are especially interesting to scientists studying nature vs nurture.

It is a myth that our physical attributes are a result of our genetics but our behavior is the result of our environment (Turkheimer, n.d.). More genetically-related persons are similar in weight, height, intelligence and even mental illness (Turkheimer, n.d.). At the same time, the environment has an effect on how our behavior is shaped eventually. Modern DNA technology has definitively answered the most sought after questions regarding nature vs nurture. However, modern DNA cannot answer all the important questions about nature versus nurture. There are very complicated issues about raising adopted twins in the same place or in different places, for example. This shows that some character traits and physical attributes are inherited, while others are learned from the adopted parents (Turkheimer, n.d.). This evidence suggests that genes work in concert with each other to determine our nature (Turkheimer, n.d.).

Have you heard about the Ambiguous Images experiment? In Category Archives: Ambiguous Images (2018) as well as a video documentary by National Geographic (2015), the role of perception in human understanding is made clear. Of course perception is not reality. Except that it reveals to psychologists the reality of different individuals. This shows how their brains process information - and the perspectives from which they understand the truth. In the real world, many people create their own respective realities based on their very poor understanding of the nature of truth. Hence, the time-tested way of arriving closer at the truth is to use facts, evidence and reason. That way, we can all agree to the objective reality.

Based on the wrong assumptions or the tricks our minds can play on us, we see in the video of the hand that is being stroked with the brush in Sweden that the subject of the research is carried along by his perception of seeing the brushed hand as his (National Geographic, 2015). This is probably because he expected his hand to be where the glove hand had been placed. "There's no question that that's my hand that, that is what you're touching, it's crazy", the subject of the research says when the brushing had ended (National Geographic, 2015, 1:57). The fact and the reality is that he could still move his right hand that had been attached to the rubber glove while believing that the hand was his (National Geographic, 2015, 1:57). Both the subject of the research and the viewer, as well as many who have commented on that video, agree that the hand was not that of the subject - a fact that is analyzed based on the evidence and on reason (National Geographic, 2015, 1:57). The fact also remains that what the subject was experiencing was his reality, though it is not real. This, therefore, makes psychological research into how the brain works very fascinating - and it will lead all of us to arrive closer at the truth.

The Ambiguous Images are equally a very fascinating exposition of the human experience - that there could be different perspectives to addressing the same situation (Category Archives: Ambiguous Images, 2018). What this means is that we should be slower to pass judgment, or at least limit our opinions to the limits of our knowledge. Interestingly the various perspectives - which one is exposed to - cannot be contested because those facts also exist. The unique thing about the hand stroking video is that the researcher did not place brush strokes on the man's hand. In the Ambiguous Images scenarios, however, one cannot just tell by looking at the photographs of the Oxford Compendium of Visual Illusions whether or not the dinosaur images, for example, were being rotated in either direction. It is only those who created that video who could report the effect they sought to create. Despite that, the issue still remains that it is the human beings who are watching the dinosaurs who can tell what they are experiencing and when. Finally, in that dinosaur video (Category Archives: Ambiguous Images, 2018), the writer tells us to put our minds to a particular perspective - and then suddenly our minds become opened to that reality and perspective (Category Archives: Ambiguous Images, 2018). This confirms the saying "the eye cannot see what the mind does not know".

When you have a sense of purpose regarding your calling in life, you tend toward choosing a vocation as a career/profession. This has concomitant effects on your physical and emotional health (Waters, 2023). Waters (2023) hence advocates a skillful vocation which thrives on your skills to serve humankind. Nursing or Caregiving is a calling; a vocation which requires skill sets from all of the various fields of human endeavor to enhance and promote human health. In conclusion, our answer to the question which forms the title of this chapter is "yes"; most people can be trained to do the same basic things. You cannot guarantee total client satisfaction, but you can at least agree in your heart that you have done the minimum that is required, the minimum that is expected of you.

8

OBEDIENCE TO INSTRUCTIONS AND WHEN TO TAKE SOLE DECISIONS BASED ON SOUND ETHICAL JUDGMENT

Isaac Ato Mensah

Barbara Vanessa Sabbi

The essence of this chapter is to raise for discussion an important decision making gray matter - professional sole decision making. Such professional sole decision making moments arise when your sole ethical judgment is required. Those occasions come and go daily in every profession when the ethical guidelines of your profession/employer cannot address some judgment calls required on the spur of the moment. Such a moment could have serious financial implications. Or they could be on the precipice of a life and death situation involving an aged person.

As former US President Abraham Lincoln once said: "You can fool all the people some of the time and you can fool some of the people all of the time but you cannot fool all the people all of the time". That was exactly the situation in Germany with Adolf Hitler. Of course not all Germans obeyed Hitler. However the fact that so many Germans obeyed sheepishly remains a concern.

Fortunately, the answer about why so many Germans followed and obeyed Hitler begins right from the immediate post-Nazi era in Germany during the Nuremberg Trials. One lasting Legacy of the Nuremberg Trials is that accused persons who tried to put the blame on superior authority as having ordered them to commit those dastardly acts of exterminating their fellow humans were told in plain language that they bore personal responsibility for their acts of omission and commission. Importantly, the Nuremberg Trials established that vicarious liability would not be extended to superiors and supervisors (Mensah, 2020). To wit, do not obey unlawful orders.

The Milgram experiment, one of the most famous experiments in psychology, has firmly established in a rather intriguing manner that many people will willingly choose to do things that will even hurt themselves (McLeod, 2017). Stanley Milgram, a professor in psychology at Yale University conducted the popular research that tried to resolve the conflict between "obedience to authority and personal conscience" (McLeod, 2017, para. 1). Milgram's work has been tested in several situations ever since. It turns out that Germans are not as cruel as one might think. Several reasons explain this.

First, there were many people who opposed Hitler from within Germany although they may have done so secretly. "The Sound of Music" movie, for example, demonstrates Captain von Trapp and the von Trapp family trying to escape Adolf Hitler's rule. Second, the fact that when the majority of Germans had the chance during and following the Nuremberg Trials, they denounced the atrocities meant that it was not in their nature to be so cruel, for, if they were, what then explains the sudden change of attitude when the Nazi regime was no longer in power? And third, if under successive German political administrations, at least since Hitler, there had been a blind obedience to authority, then one could argue strongly that a trend of unusually cruel behavior has been established. However, the historical record rather shows that Germans have been expanding their freedom frontiers since Adolf Hitler.

Haslam, Reicher and Millard (2015) revisited the obedience to authority research. Indeed Haslam, Reicher and Millard (2015) used Immersive Digital Realism (IDR), an ethically sound research technique, to gauge the extent to which 14 actors who were subjects of their research would obey unlawful orders. The researchers observed that all participants were willing to give shocks greater than 150 Volts, just as in the original Stanley Milgram experiment. However, when the participants were told that they had no choice in the matter even as the voltages were increased, they all refused to continue cooperating with the research team, clearly suggesting that human beings and particularly the Germans had a choice - a choice to walk away from Hitler and not obey unlawful orders. As Saint Augustine of Hippo has explained, the greatest problem God has given to humankind is the problem of free choice. We humans are always free to choose what is good or bad for us; what we will do and what we will not do; and the freedom to choose whether or not we want to stay in the game and suffer the consequences of our actions. The failure to recognise the situation the Germans faced is, therefore, a clear case of cognitive bias which psychologists have christened the Fundamental Attribution Error (FAE).

Indeed in a later research, Haslam and Reicher (2018) concluded that social identities - be they German, American, or whatever chains we put ourselves in - apologies Jean-Jacques Rousseau - are not the determinants of our actions (Deneys-Tunney, 2012). This clearly removes the idea that humans are mechanistic robots (Deneys-Tunney, 2012). It is important, however, to recognize that humankind's everyday communication is influenced - not determined - by the social roles we endorse and the chains we leash ourselves with (Jouffre & Croizet, 2016). Burger (2014) has identified four characteristic features that made the original Milgram experiment a success, including the fact that the voltages were increased gradually. Indeed, the historical record has it that Hitler did not immediately come onto the scene as a dictator. Perhaps, if he had, many Germans would have immediately opposed him, leaving no room for any Nazi propaganda to fester.

"In fact, [Fundamental Attribution Error, or FAE] is at the root of any misunderstanding in which human motivations have the potential to be misinterpreted" (Healy, 2017, para. 9). Healy (2017), therefore, suggests that humans should develop more emotional intelligence to overcome FAE, which is so common among humankind's cognitive biases.

FAE has been described as the tendency for us humans to explain the reason for other people's behavior as due to their personality traits rather than a factor of the situation they may find themselves in, while at the same time downplaying the same effect in our own behavior (Moran et al., 2014). FAE has been found to be common across cultures (Lee & Fiore, 2020). This context should help us do our job of safeguarding the aged by being circumspect in our judgment of issues at the workplace. Above all, safeguarding the aged requires both passion and compassion. When you work in a hospice, for example, - a place where terminally ill persons are on admission - you cannot help but develop compassion for the aged, sick and dying. In a hospice, the scent in the environment may not be that pleasant for obvious reasons. Now if you work here for at least 12 months, you may become more philosophical about the meaning of life and the end of life. You may then develop more passion and compassion for your work.

CASE STUDY:

RESIDENT X NEEDS EXTRA CARE

Resident X is the typical case of someone who is delicate when it comes to food. She lives in a nursing care home. She is well informed of her right to refuse whatever treatment or caregiving she is uncomfortable with. She has been a client in a care facility for more than a year. She is living with dementia and other comorbidities. She does not sleep at night; she just keeps walking. She will not allow you to change her pads or otherwise clean her up when she has soiled herself. She will walk around the whole place within the building. When it is time for meals, she will not eat. When she is fed, she will reject the food, throw it up.

She uses vulgar words, and has an acerbic tongue. In short she is a difficult customer. She even fights the staff. For example, she will condemn the food as being only good for dogs or cats. You cannot change his clothes until she herself is willing and has calmed down. It is simply too difficult on the care workers such that they often need to fall on the nurses for assistance. You will be required to use all the skills you can muster to enlist her cooperation. Often you will come to your wits end. You will even coax her into eating or getting something done for herself, all to no avail; she will insult you and sack you from her presence. Yet you have to do your job. In the western world, where nursing care homes are well established, when a resident refuses care, they are within their rights so to do so you have to just leave them. But you can't leave them; you have to do your job. In any case, if you leave them alone, a report will be made against you because you left the resident unattended. In such cases the routine is to go report to the nurse. Sometimes the Nurses have some meds that they give to such patients to make them calm down. Yet more often than not, it never seems to work. Just two days earlier it was better; she even allowed the care team to attend to her and everyone was on board - excited to help. Yesterday, she went on an upward swing again. She was sitting at a dining table with someone's juice and water right in front of her. She was about to drink it when she was prompted that what she was taking was for someone else. Then she flipped. You can imagine all the expletives she used and physical harm she was about to cause to the staff attending to her.

It is fairly routine for her to slap the staff. The staff believe strongly that even though she has dementia, she is quite aware of everything happening around her. This is because she will tell you flatly that you cannot do anything to her because you get paid to work. She will warn you in no uncertain terms that if you do anything to her she will report you. When she says that you know you cannot do anything to her and the authorities will not do anything about it because you signed up for that job. You took the water out in the presence of other residents because it does not belong to her and warned her that she cannot hit you. Then the other residents told her in unison that she could not do that because the water did not belong to her. You then supplied her with a new bottle of water. Then you realized suddenly that maybe you should have supplied the new bottle of water before removing the old one.

That's one skill you failed to utilize on the spur of the moment. As you keep working, you keep learning. However, what will you do differently? In all of this, never forget to document whatever happens because the Nurses will need that record to decide what to do next. When the documentation is in place, the Nurses can report it to the families of the residents who can talk to them. With all the documentation intact, you can save yourself a lot of trouble.

9

CAREGIVING BY RELATIVES AS SAFEGUARDING - A CULTURAL WEALTH PERSPECTIVE

Isaac Ato Mensah

Barbara Vanessa Sabbi

In many parts of the world, the role of relatives as caregivers is an age-old tradition. Caregiving has held its own even as orthodox medicine has not seen much penetration in many rural communities around the world. Even among the controversial Trokosi practitioners in Ghana, caregiving at home is the dominant theme (Mensah, 2023).

All human beings are born equal and thus have universal needs such as dignity and inclusion for which reason they may exhibit resistant capital until they have achieved those dreams (Hansen, 2021). Therefore in going about our routine activities we all seek to maximize the resources we have and naturally exchange them for other goods and services so that we can fend for ourselves. The extent to which human beings can exchange more of the resources they have will determine how rich or poor they become, thus emphasizing their cultural wealth prowess (Hansen, 2021).

Tara J. Yoso defined cultural wealth as "an array of knowledge, skills, strengths and experiences that are learned and shared by people of color and marginalized groups; the values and behaviors that are nurtured through culture work together to create a way of knowing and being" (Hansen, 2021, para. 2).

The French sociologist Pierre Bourdieu's cultural capital model, meanwhile, argues that our tastes depend on the social groups within which we fall. "Bourdieu defined cultural capital as 'familiarity with the legitimate culture within a society'; what we might call 'high culture'" (Cultural Learning Alliance, 2019, para. 3). These tastes tend to be uniform across social groups. Since people of one cultural group tend to have the same cultural capital more or less, they will more likely have a higher purchasing power when it comes to bargaining for goods and services than another group with a lower cultural capital (Then & Now, 2019; Cultural Learning Alliance, 2019). By way of analogy, people who enjoy Bach's classical Music will likely have a higher purchasing power than those who attend LL Cool J's rap music concerts (Then & Now, 2019). This is because the lovers of rap music usually have a street culture background, come from low income families, treasure graffiti which is a sign of a push back or resistance embarked upon by the lower echelons of the society and tend to treasure DJs and MCs (Then & Now, 2019).

Not so with classical music lovers who tend to spend a lot of time examining classical music compositions, read books about classical music, pay more to attend classical music concerts and wear suits while attending such opera shows. For crying out loud one needs only a T-shirt, a pair of jeans and trainers to attend a rap music show. The Chale Wote Festival held annually in James Town, Accra, is a case in point (Nimo, 2022). It is an art festival designed primarily for those who wear bathroom slippers in their daily commutes; the man on the street. These are the downtrodden; or if you prefer, the streetwise (Nimo, 2022). We can, therefore, say as a rule of thumb that those lovers of classical music will more likely have a higher income status and a higher status in society generally than rap music lovers. This has implications for which communities of people can afford assisted living services or nursing care home services now.

Therefore, while cultural capital is available to everyone, some people have a higher purchasing power with their cultural capital than others. In short knowledge is power and "cultural capital engaged over lifetimes is often more powerful than economic capital" (Then & Now, 2019, 14:40). The Ga-Dangme people of Greater Accra, Ghana, for example, have their own unique cultural capital, and they need more radio frequencies, for example, to enable them communicate that power so that they can uplift their people from mass poverty. Such a medium will empower them to challenge almost immediately, all stereotypes against them such as, the Ga language is loud and aggressive which deters interest in learning the language. These stereotypes are foisted upon them while they are a minority ethnic group in their own indigenous/ancestral home.

It is an undeniable fact that the Ga and Dangme people have suffered a lot of disrespect on account of their collective relatively less cultural capital. But all is not lost. Yosso's cultural wealth model espouses the power of the wealth that people from African and Latino backgrounds, for example, bring to work, classroom and other environments where they are considered minorities (Yosso, 2005). Yosso's cultural wealth model includes six types of capital by which the marginalized may show resilience and thrive in difficult circumstances (Yosso, 2005).

For instance, Yosso talks about familial capital which refers to the extended family and community network connections that immigrants can draw upon for collective empowerment (Hansen, 2021; Yosso, 2005). People from West African backgrounds, for example, often have great storytelling abilities which we have acquired by associating with the elderly who are the custodians of such folklore as Brer Rabbit and Kweku Ananse (Mensah, 2023). Such storytelling abilities are referred to as linguistic capital and could be used for behavior change communication when the moral import of those stories are impressed upon our people through radio broadcasting, for example, such as the Ga are advocating for (Hansen, 2021; Yosso, 2005).

In Outliers, Malcolm Gladwell, famously described the Roseto effect as a family of grandparents, parents, uncles, cousins and children who lived in family clusters in rural Pennsylvania and worked the land through drudgery up and down the hills day and night. Such a hard life helped them build resistance, and no one under age 65 was known to have a heart disease even when the U.S. was experiencing a heart disease epidemic at the time (Gladwell, 2008). These were illiterate Italian migrants who spoke mainly Italian in a community dominated by mainly English speakers. Thus they showed a lot of cultural capital to offer America and the world, they being a marginalized community who were demonstrating aspirational capital, social capital, familial capital, and resistant capital (Hansen, 2021; Gladwell, 2008). Many immigrant communities also possess a lot of cultural wealth/cultural capital which they can use to lift their kith and kin out of poverty, squalor and disease (Hansen, 2021; Gladwell, 2008; Yosso, 2005).

10

CAN POPULATION HEALTH ISSUES TEACH US ABOUT SAFEGUARDING THE AGED?

Isaac Ato Mensah

Population health could be defined as a holistic conceptualization of health that starts with the traditional public health roles of doing away with diseases and injuries, and then extends into health promotion and longevity, thus engendering a multisectoral approach to improve the health of a specific population usually defined by location and other demographics.

The wide range of issues that influence population health include the environment of course, social mobility, income status, type of employment, access to health services, in-group and out-group stereotyping, type of housing and accommodation and what have you. All such issues "revolve around three major pillars — human health, environmental resilience and social and economic equity — that affect the lives of billions of people around the world" (University of Washington, n.d., para. 3). Given this context, the aged persons in the respective counties and districts chosen are a defined population. They could thus benefit from population health planning.

A study of the medical geography of Ghana, or whichever jurisdiction you find yourself in, will, no doubt, reveal a lot about the population health profile of your community. In other words, there are several important teaching points that when properly understood will seriously impact population health practices. Take the Krobo people of Ghana, for example. Oral history from several reliable sources reveal why Krobo women are perceived as promiscuous and HIV is widely assumed to be high among them. Let us begin the search by looking at the family history of

Dr Edward Narh, President of Narh-Bita College and founder of Narh-Bita Hospital. He is an indigene of Manya Krobo with boundaries in the Greater Accra Region and Eastern Region of Ghana. He narrates that when the Basel Missionaries settled in Krobo land, the early converts included one adult male by name Narh, who was his grandfather. This Narh was ostracized by his own extended family for accepting Christianity. As a result, the ostracized Narh eventually established a new family with his wife Mamle Djange in a different part of the town. Since there were two men by name Narh in the original extended family, Dr Narh's ancestor became Narh Beta, as in alpha, beta, theta, to differentiate the Narh who was the alpha or elder. This was eventually simplified as Narh-Bita so that no one will mispronounce the name as Narh Better.

It is not uncommon to find such ostracisation in many communities around the world. One can only imagine what will happen to females who may get ostracized among the early converts. Once they live away from home, then it becomes virtually impossible to undergo the Dipo rituals which are the traditional puberty rites for adolescent girls. Puberty rites are a celebration of virginity. Over time, all the women who could not undertake the rites as a result of such departures from their ancestral homes could easily become labeled as promiscuous. And of course promiscuity is a sexually risky behavior which has implications for contracting sexually transmitted infections including the Human Immunodeficiency Virus (HIV). The Krobo people are mainly populous in and around Koforidua, the regional capital under which their homeland falls. Many of them are also in the Greater Accra Region within which part of their homeland falls. Thus, the higher than average HIV infections for towns and communities around Accra and Koforidua are often popularly attributed mainly to the Krobo in street talk.

We have thus given the historical antecedents to show evidence that where a higher prevalence among people living around Koforidua and Accra exists, ostracisation from traditional mores, norms and culture could be a predisposing factor. The stereotyping is almost hardwired in the human brain especially when they cannot help but see themselves in terms of their in-groups and outgroups in virtually any social context.

Moving forward, in Ghana today, as in many other nation-states, will it be so easy to identify so-called pure breeds of ethnic people? Given this antecedent of the Krobo people, have they not suffered enough historical trauma for which they need special population health planning and safeguarding of their aged, especially the Krobo women? How difficult will it be to identify all such persons who migrated away from their ancestral/spiritual homelands as a result of such unfortunate situations? Please try identifying such historical events in your family/community and how it may have affected your health and wellbeing today. Not all such experiences end up in traumatic conditions. Some persons and communities are able to overcome their horrid past, thereby developing resistant capital as an important cultural wealth contribution to the growth of humanity (Hansen, 2021; Durham & Webb, 2014).

11

SOCIALISATION, HISTORICAL TRAUMA AND CAREGIVING

Barbara Vanessa Sabbi

Isaac Ato Mensah

The ADDRESSING model "is a framework that facilitates recognition and understanding of the complexities of individual identity" (Ohio University, n.d., para. 1). According to Hays, "consideration of **a**ge, **d**evelopmental **d**isabilities, acquired **d**isabilities, **r**eligion, **e**thnicity, **s**exual orientation, **s**ocioeconomic status, **i**ndigenous group membership, **n**ationality, and **g**ender contribute to a complete understanding of cultural identity. Each factor can help researchers understand underrepresented groups and oppressive forces (Ohio University, n.d., para. 1). Please observe how the highlighted letters in the quote above spell the acronym ADDRESSING. This model is, therefore, appropriate for understanding a whole lifetime of events, especially historical trauma, as it relates to some chronic conditions which a Caregiver - make that your aged relative - may experience.

The idea that not only physiological factors, but environmental factors also do cause stress is common knowledge (University of Washington, n.d.). Socio-cultural factors, a subset of environmental factors that cause stress and impact health include incomes, the work environment, discrimination, pollution - to name just a few (University of Washington, n.d.). A further impetus to this observation has been discussed by Harris (2014) in a Ted Talk video wherein it is explained that childhood trauma can affect human hormones. Dr. Harris (2014) explains that in later life, childhood trauma can cause chronic diseases (lifelong illnesses such as heart problems). This is the predicament of many First Nations and Native American people, for example, who were taught to acquiesce and conform to dehumanization through a forced boarding school system (alchemicalmedia, 2013).

In the Unseen Tears video, the sadness, disappointment, shock and dismay about obnoxiously forcing people to speak English and be civilized according to someone else's culture is clear (alchemicalmedia, 2013; Emotion & Feeling, n.d.). The children were conformists, much like many of us in our childhood; they succumbed to whatever was being taught them. They sang the song "One little, two little, three little Indians" - a song that derided them (alchemicalmedia, 2013). This story and song resonate with many people because growing up in the British colonial system and its horrible legacy, many people also used to sing songs such as, "I am a donkey, donkey follow me". These songs were used by the teachers when they had some corporal punishment lined up for the students. Such corporal punishment included holding your ears and doing squat and stand. Immediately a student was fished out, their colleagues would start teasing with the song. Is it not any wonder yet, that Medical Doctors are not trained to handle such cases? Dr Harris, therefore, believes that medical care should be holistic, thus the relevance of the ADDRESSING model (Ohio University, n.d.).

Harris (2014) presents a summary of a famous research - The Adverse Childhood Experiences Study (ACE) - which was done by surveying 17500 adults. The survey covered childhood experiences. The researchers then drew a correlation between those experiences and health outcomes. The research was carried out by the Centers for Disease Control and the Kaiser

Permanente health care organization in California. When Dr. Harris worked in rural San Francisco, California and so many children (patients) were referred to her for Attention Deficit Hyperactivity Disorder (ADHD), she decided to probe further. Then a colleague introduced her to the research on ACEs which shows there is "a 20 year difference in life expectancy" among those who have experienced childhood trauma and those who have not (Harris, 2014, 0:28). The problem of childhood trauma is so serious that in later life, for example, the prefrontal cortex that controls emotions is inhibited. She discovered that Ischemic heart disease, for example, is indicative of childhood trauma.

In the original study by the Centers for Disease Control and the Kaiser Permanente health care organization in California, an Adverse Childhood Experience (ACE) was defined as three "specific kinds of adversity children faced in the home environment—various forms of physical and emotional abuse, neglect, and household dysfunction" (Harvard University, n.d., para. 1). "There is a powerful, persistent correlation between [four or] more ACEs experienced and the greater the chance of poor outcomes later in life, including dramatically increased risk of heart disease, diabetes, obesity, depression, substance abuse, smoking, poor academic achievement, time out of work, and early death" (Harvard University, n.d., para. 1). For persons with an ACE score of four or more, "their relative risk of chronic obstructive pulmonary disease was two-and-a-half times that of someone with an ACE score of zero" (Harris, 2014, 10:02).

A panoramic perspective means that all shades of opinion across the world or different dimensions are being considered. Hence, we take the liberty to share perspectives from across the world. Durham and Webb (2014), Medical

Doctors with experiential knowledge of working with historical trauma have explained that not all families live with the burden of trauma. "Some families are more resilient than others and are able to acknowledge the past while looking toward the future" (Durham & Webb, 2014, p. 1). The challenge then is to treat patients by looking at their generational history in terms of war, deprivation, slavery, substance abuse, etc., in addressing whatever issues may be presented at the clinic (Substance Abuse and Mental Health Services Administration, 2009).

Meanwhile, there is enough evidence that diet affects health and longevity, and the ability to function well on a task (Harding et al., 2015). Long periods of poor dieting therefore can lead to untold health problems in future. Simply put, historical trauma refers to long periods of deprivation or forced control of another group of people which create untold consequences among generations of those people in many aspects of their lives. When historical trauma is not resolved people will live with it all their lives. Durham and Webb (2014) suggest that First Nations people and holocaust survivors, for example, are likely to carry the effects of pain from historical trauma. Therefore, "understanding more about historical trauma and how it impacts families will hopefully add a new dimension to the perspective through which we view not only our patients and their families, but also ourselves" (Durham & Webb, 2014, p. 6).

Let us mention in passing some identifiable issues which could cause historical trauma for the indigenous people of the Western North Region, Upper West Region, Upper East Region, and Savannah Region. First, Western North. This area has several mining companies operating there. There have been numerous reports of land degradation and pollution of rivers by mining companies who simply allow cyanide to flow into the rivers - all to no avail. And now Galamsey - an illegal mining that diverts the course of river bodies and turns the water brownish - is the new normal in the districts of the Western North Region. The Upper West Region, Upper East Region and Savannah Region have suffered from the collateral damage occasioned by the annual spillage of the Bagri Dam from the neighboring country of Burkina Faso, Cerebrospinal Meningitis (CSM) and bloody nostrils as a result of the harsh annual Harmattan dry and dusty winds, to name but a few. Eventually, these things do affect people and their progeny for generations. The frequent inter-ethnic conflicts also have implications for migration (Kwansa, 2020). The irrigation dams in these communities, including in Bongo in the Upper East Region, are evidence that "large water bodies impact year-round carriage of submicroscopic parasites and sustain *Plasmodium* transmission" (Kyei-Baffour et al., 2020, para. 1). What issues can you identify within your community that you think can impact the population health of your people?

Given such envisaged problems which can affect even an unborn child, the Apgar assessment will come in handy (Harris, 2014; Lally & Valentine-French, 2020). The Apgar assessment assesses a neonate's circumstances using five parameters namely, the heart rate, breathing, tone of muscle, color, and reflex response (known as the Babinski reflex). The Neonatal Behavioral Assessment Scale (NBAS) is also another option (Lally & Valentine-French, 2020). We can use these parameters to look at The Navajo Nation or any other population of your choice which has suffered historical trauma, and then document their sufferings (Chinle Chapter Government, 2020). At long last, Belgium, through King Philippe, has admitted that they did wrong in their colonial handling of the Congo (Ilunga, 2022). During colonialism, an estimated 10 million Congolese died or disappeared (Ilunga, 2022). Some Congolese reportedly had their hands and feet cut off (Ilunga, 2022). All this is enough evidence that these persons and their progeny have suffered historical trauma (Harris, 2014; alchemicalmedia, 2013). In recognition of the historical abuse and in the spirit of addressing historical trauma, the Navajo Area Indian Health Service, for example, will have to ensure individuals eat healthily and engage in relevant exercises that help combat obesity-related health problems, irrespective of an individual's financial status (Chinle Chapter Government, 2020). This is possible through local government funding.

Obesity is the number one cause of mortality in the Chinle community. US data shows that the median income of the Chinle community is about US$30,000 (Chinle Chapter Government, 2020; United States Census Bureau, n.d.). All told, the dangerous health consequences of poor eating coupled with a sedentary lifestyle is detrimental to human health (Chinle Chapter Government, 2020). Those who overcome such trauma have important lessons for all humankind. Yosso's cultural wealth model highlights the power of the wealth of people from minority backgrounds (Yosso, 2005). Yosso's cultural wealth model includes six different types of capital by which human beings overcome challenges (Yosso, 2005). This is the real learning moment for us: That all those things we were subjected to as children were wrong. Thus has the healing process begun, for, the awareness of the knowledge itself is empowering. Quite frankly, for a long time, we've been wondering why those who committed such childhood offenses against their kith and kin never apologized, but rather justified it.

This matter resonates well with a lot of people because in many parts of the world such as Ghana, Togo, Benin, Nigeria, India, Ceylon, Malaysia, China, Bangladesh, Chile, Bolivia - you name it - carbohydrate-based diets are the usual family's main staple foods. And we choose these primarily because we cannot afford the more nutritious diets such as mediterranean diets (Hardman et al., 2015). Meanwhile, all this is still happening even in the face of the evidence that diet affects health, longevity, and the ability to function well on a task (Harding et al., 2015).

This final point is important because for a long time, many people have been trying to figure out the reasons for what happened to them. But now, thanks to the collaborative research effort that produced this book, we have a scholarly reference in the ADDRESSING model which offers "a complete understanding of cultural identity" - of who we are and have become (Ohio University, n.d., para. 1). Many people have kept a good balance between working, schooling, family life and socializing without becoming social misfits or developing mental problems. In other words, they have developed resilience to historical trauma (Durham & Webb, 2014).

Alternatively, the Bronfenbrenner model also explains the concept of time dimension in understanding a person's socialization (Oswalt, n.d.). "Bronfenbrenner's final level is the macrosystem, which is the largest and most diverse set of people and things in a person's environment. The macrosystem has a great influence over the child. The macrosystem includes things such as the relative freedoms permitted by your national government, cultural values, the economy, wars, etc. These things can also affect a child either positively or negatively" (Oswalt, n.d., para. 4). How have you been affected by historical trauma?

12

THE PROSPECTUS FOR THE PROPOSED ASSISTED LIVING PROGRAM FOR KING COUNTY IN WASHINGTON STATE, USA.

PART I: JUSTIFICATION OF THE NEED FOR A COUNTY SPONSORED PROGRAM

Edem Ahiati

Isaac Ato Mensah

We compare data from four of the selected regions of Ghana to King County in Washington State in the US and propose assisted living programs for both jurisdictions. Both jurisdictions are based on unique population characteristics and health needs in those places. This approach is justified by adopting a similar comparative method of analysis used by Sir Jack Goody, a renowned British anthropologist. Goody compared the societies of ancient Greece to those of the northern parts of modern Ghana and established links between different civilisations and the processes of change (Mensah, 2018).

THE NEED FOR ASSISTED DAILY LIVING

People are getting older in the U.S., and with old age comes lifestyle diseases and often solitary lives when older people have reached the empty nest stage of life (American Association of Retired Persons [AARP], 2020). Issues of historical trauma are known to be indicative of lifetime diseases including chronic diseases which develop in later life (Harris, 2014). People who have suffered historical trauma and now live alone at home while suffering comorbidities must, therefore, be going through a lot more difficulty. Income inequality is 4.7% for King County, 4.5% for Washington State and 3.7% for the top U.S. performers and is a social determinant of health (County Health Rankings and Roadmap, n.d.).

Air pollution is equally worse for King County compared to Washington State and the top U.S. performers (County Health Rankings and Roadmap, n.d.). Of course, it goes without saying that this has an effect when one is counting social determinants of health even though pollution is usually considered a matter that affects the physical environment (County Health Rankings and Roadmap, n.d.).

The picture is equally stark when one looks at the data for severe housing problems, that is, 18% for King County, 18% for Washington State, and 9% for the top U.S. performers (County Health Rankings and Roadmap, n.d.). Using the 2019 population estimate for King County of 2,253,000 this means a whopping 405,540 people in King County have severe housing problems (United States Census Bureau, n.d.).

In terms of the uninsured population, King County is basically at par with the best: 6% for King County, 7% for Washington State, and 6% for the top U.S. performers (County Health Rankings and Roadmap, n.d.). This means some of the vulnerable people of King County and their surrounding neighbors within Washington State need Medicare and Medicaid (County Health Rankings and Roadmap, n.d.). Adult obesity is 22% for King County, 28% for Washington State, and 26% for the top U.S. performers. This is indicative of impending or current chronic diseases (County Health Rankings and Roadmap, n.d.). Even though the percentage of people with adult obesity is slightly better for King County, in terms of the attendant disease burden, the figure leaves much to be desired (County Health Rankings and Roadmap, n.d.). These statistics present us with a continuous stream of present and future adults aged 65 and older who will constantly have to live with comorbidities and geriatric healthcare solutions including help with assisted living (County Health Rankings and Roadmap, n.d.; AARP, 2020).

PROPOSED INNOVATIVE SOLUTION

The innovative solution more directly addresses the domain of risk prevention and reduction and when people who need assisted living are injured at home, the health and financial ramifications may become a nightmare. Relatives may lose working hours in order to give more attention to the injured elderly. This is all preventable when taxpayers' dollars are spent to promote assisted living.

The solution is a policy reform that offers restorative justice for people who may have suffered years of historical trauma. The fact that all persons 65 years and older who have the need for assisted living should qualify for county support under this proposed King County Assisted Living Program is a way of giving back to the elderly for their many years of work for the society. The fact is a potential 7% of the population will be impacted (County Health Rankings and Roadmap, n.d.). Among these are elderly people who may have suffered historical trauma, but who will now receive financial or human resource support for assisted living under the proposed King County Assisted Living Program (KCALP). This shows a shift from volume-based care to value-based care (County Health Rankings and Roadmap, n.d.).

This solution, the proposed King County Assisted Living Program (KCALP), promotes value-based care such that no persons who need assisted living will be left behind (American Hospital Association, 2014). Whole-person care and person-centered care are recurrent themes of the second wave of healthcare transformation in the United States (American Hospital Association, 2014). Indigenous people, especially people who have suffered historical trauma, generally, have obviously been let down by society (Harvard University, n.d.; Harris, 2014; alchemicalmedia, 2013). Once the healthcare system failed in supporting them when they were young, now the King County Government should not miss this opportunity to support elderly indigenous people through the assisted living program (Harris, 2014; alchemicalmedia, 2013).

This proposed assisted living program offers more efficiency in caregiving since the subscribers can either stay at home or receive care through an assisted living facility. More likely, the clients/subscribers who are the direct oldies in need of assisted living will not feel emotionally separated from their loved ones when they are at home receiving the needed care. Those who may opt to go to long term care facilities may, however, feel emotionally separated when they go into a care facility under the KCALP.

VALUE PROPOSITION

The King County Assisted Living Program will promote assisted living, which is an essential part of value-based care (American Hospital Association, 2014). This will show that the King County Government is committed to addressing the problems created by historical trauma, especially trauma suffered by indigenous peoples (Harris, 2014; Harvard University, n.d.; alchemicalmedia, 2013). Seattle, Washington is the largest city in King County with about 750,000 residents as of 2020. King County itself has about 2.2 million people. The aged, that is, people 65 years and older among them constitute 13 percent of that 2.2 million, namely, 286,000 people (American Association of Retired Persons [AARP], 2020).

Aged people who experience falls at home are a serious health problem (AARP, 2020; Hatcher, 2020; Bu et al., 2020). The proposed King County Assisted Living Program will, therefore, help to minimize that risk. This gray matter supports a mixture of home-based assisted living or institution-based assisted living, depending on client/subscriber preferences. This is based on the research evidence that alternative care locations versus home care hold heterogeneous outcomes of quality of care for the elderly (Boland et al., 2017).

The research by Boland et al. (2017, para. 3) showed that "Three hundred and forty studies [involving] 271,660 participants were synthesized. "The categories of comparisons included: home with support versus independent living at home ($n = 11$ reviews), home care versus institutional care ($n = 3$ reviews), and rehabilitation at home versus conventional rehabilitation services ($n = 7$ reviews). Two reviews had data relevant to two categories. Most reviews favored home with support [for] independent living at home. Findings comparing home care to institutional care were mixed. Most reviews found no differences in health outcomes between rehabilitation at home versus conventional rehabilitation services" (Boland et al., 2017, para. 3). Assisted living, being implemented by the King County Government will improve the population health profile of King County when it is implemented over time. This is because many of the seniors will otherwise have no means of getting the wherewithal to fully fund the cost of assisted living, estimated at about USD3000 monthly (Devaney, n.d.).

13

THE PROSPECTUS FOR THE PROPOSED ASSISTED LIVING PROGRAM FOR KING COUNTY IN WASHINGTON STATE, USA

PART II: STAKEHOLDER ANALYSIS

Edem Ahiati

Isaac Ato Mensah

Three internal stakeholders who will be most impacted by the need for the proposed King County Assisted Living Program, in our estimation, are: 1) King County Council, 2) King County Board of Health, and 3) King County Auditor.

The individuals identified in the list of internal stakeholders will feel a direct responsibility to fail or succeed. If the program succeeds, they will feel more empowered to continue and improve it. If on the other hand, the town hall meetings fail or there is lack of consensus about how to proceed, these stakeholders may come under pressure to account for a waste of the resources used in promoting the proposed assisted living program.

INTERNAL STAKEHOLDERS

1) King County Council, 2) King County Board of Health, and 3) King County Auditor.

The individuals identified in the list of internal stakeholders will feel a direct responsibility to fail or succeed. If the program succeeds, they will feel more empowered to continue and improve it. If on the other hand, the town hall meetings fail or there is lack of consensus about how to proceed, these stakeholders may come under pressure to account for a possible waste of resources used in promoting the proposed assisted living program.

External Stakeholders: 1) persons in need of assisted living together with their relatives, 2) community colleges and other training institutions that may train students under our proposed King County Assisted Living program, 3) integrated delivery systems which already offer assisted living services in Washington State.

These external stakeholders are likely to invest considerable resources into the proposed assisted living program, expecting it to succeed. If all goes well, they will likely feel that they have made a good investment. On the other hand, if the program fails or is discontinued within the foreseeable future, these external stakeholders will likely feel they have wasted their resources in the lobbying and advocacy process. Elderly persons will likely become more empowered and more trusting of the government, policymakers and elected officials. This is because they may begin to see that legislation has been passed to support the quality of assisted living programs. They will also more likely perceive that the quality of assisted living is improving.

EXTERNAL STAKEHOLDERS

Three external stakeholders who will be most impacted by the need for the proposed King County Assisted Living Program, in our estimation, are: 1) persons in need of assisted living, together with their relatives, 2) community colleges and other training institutions that may train students under the proposed King County Assisted Living Program, and 3) integrated delivery systems which already offer assisted living services in Washington State. These external stakeholders are likely to invest considerable resources into the proposed assisted living program, expecting it to succeed. If all goes well, they will have made a good investment. On the other hand, if the program fails or is discontinued within the foreseeable future, the external stakeholders will feel they have wasted their resources in planning and training for such a program. The community of elderly persons will likely become more empowered and more trusting of the government, policymakers and elected officials since they will begin to see that legislation has been made to support assisted living programs. They will also see and feel that the quality of assisted living is improving.

UNIQUENESS

The innovative solution more directly addresses the domain of risk prevention and reduction, for, when people who need assisted living are injured at home, the health and financial ramifications may become a logistical nightmare (Devaney, n.d.; Hatcher, 2020). This is because relatives may lose working hours in order to give more attention to the elderly. This is preventable when taxpayers' dollars are spent to support assisted living. The solution is a policy reform that offers restorative justice for people who may have suffered years of historical trauma (Harris, 2014). The fact that all persons of age 65 and older who need assisted living will be eligible is a way of giving back to senior citizens for their many years of work for the society. The fact that a potential 7% of the population will be impacted and these elderly people will now receive financial or human resource support for assisted living shows a shift from volume-based care to value-based care (County Health Rankings and Roadmap, n.d.; American Hospital Association, 2014).

This solution integrates healthcare in a comprehensive fashion because no persons who need assisted living will be left behind. Whole-person care and person-centered care are recurrent themes of the second wave of healthcare transformation in the United States (American Hospital Association, 2014). Indigenous people and people who have suffered historical trauma generally have been let down by society (Harris, 2014). Once the healthcare system failed in supporting them when they were younger, the King County Government should not miss this opportunity to give such persons dignified care through assisted living (Harris, 2014).

Assisted living offers more efficiency in caregiving since the patients will stay in their homes and receive care. This will reduce the cost of logistics spent in caring for the patient (Hatcher, 2020). At the same time, the patients/residents will not feel much emotional loss as they will be with their loved ones at home (Devaney, n.d.). The proposed King County Assisted Living Program is being proposed as a sustaining innovation that builds on the concept of assisted living (Christensen et al., 2015). This solution is a sustaining innovation because it builds on the concepts of assisted living, either at home or at an assisted living facility (Christensen et al., 2015). Assisted living programs are already being implemented throughout the United States and are, therefore, not new (Devaney, n.d.; Hatcher, 2020). In America, by 2015, there were about 4.7 million elderly people taking advantage of home-health care, 730,000 opting for assisted living, while 1.4 million people were in nursing homes where trained personnel are ever present to attend to their needs (Neufeld, 2017). America has roughly 16,000 nursing care homes with a total bed capacity of 1.8 million (Neufeld, 2017).

OPTIMIZATION OF VALUE-BASED CARE AND PATIENT-CENTERED CARE

Prospective clients who need help with assisted living in their own homes will register with the King County Assisted Living Program, and the service will be brought to their doorstep. This will surely be counted by every stakeholder in healthcare as patient-centered care and will contribute to measurable improvements in patient-centered health and well-being because the numbers of people who will benefit can be counted (American Hospital Association, 2014). This is one of the main goals of the second curve of health care in the U.S., that is, patient-centered care, which is considered a part of value-based care (American Hospital Association, 2014; Health Research and Educational Trust, 2013). This solution optimizes value-based care (American Hospital Association, 2014).

The perception that the King County Government will be supporting direct care of patients will be very empowering, and hopefully get the support of indigenous communities. The indigenous communities are expected to help by agreeing to register their relatives who may need help with assisted living. The operational efficiency of this proposed assisted living program will be strong because King County will begin to directly enumerate all those who need assisted living. It is based on the proposed register that King County can accurately determine how many students it will sponsor each year to undergo training in assisted living at designated community colleges.

The average cost of care charged by care homes who offer assisted living services, estimated at USD3000, could be used as the estimated cost per annum per resident (Devaney, n.d.). The county will subsidize that amount by paying a third of that, viz, USD1000. This figure of USD1000, multiplied by the number of approved clients/subscribers will be the annual cost of care for elders who need assisted living. This helps achieve the goals of the second curve of healthcare in the U.S., namely value-based care (American Hospital Association, 2014; Health Research and Educational Trust, 2013). This solution, therefore, optimizes value-based care (American Hospital Association, 2014). With such a provision made, value-based care will be offered to more people who need assisted living (American Hospital Association, 2014; AARP, 2020). These indigenous communities are expected to provide expertise to enrich the program by sharing ideas on how adults can cope with the challenges of living alone.

Assisted living homes somewhat break social connections and family bonds for those who already enjoy a family bond at home judging by the fact that many many clients want to choose a facility close to where they stay, have stayed before and or where their close relatives stay (Devaney, n.d.). Those who prefer assisted living facilities will be offered the same amount of USD1,000. For people who have suffered historical abuse, being taken to nursing homes without their loved ones present may only appear to be a second dose of the obnoxious boarding school system which tried to change the worldview of indigenous children (alchemicalmedia, 2013).

The literature further tells us that "Seniors don't normally travel very far when searching for an assisted living home. In most cases, it's close to where they last resided, or where one of their children lives" (Devaney, n.d., para. 28). The implication is that running assisted living programs from the homes of the clients/subscribers is an ideal solution. Some trained caregivers living in King County who agree to care for their elderly relatives, could view the program as a working-from-home part-time employment. When the community engagement promotional campaigns including town hall meetings are done right, many people will eventually more likely believe in this proposed program.

"In Washington state, at the first U.S. nursing home with a known Covid-19 outbreak, federal officials determined that the virus had spread, in part, through staff members who worked in multiple facilities — a common practice given the paltry pay and limited benefits for direct caregivers, most of whom are people of color" (Khimm, 2021, para. 12). Thus is a further justification given for the proposed King County Assisted Living Program. This is further evidence that the suggestion by Coe (2021) that the Community Health Nurses who visit several homes a day should be given further training to attend to the aged in Ghana did not consider the risk of cross infection.

14

THE PROSPECTUS FOR THE PROPOSED ASSISTED LIVING PROGRAM FOR KING COUNTY IN WASHINGTON STATE, USA

PART III: IMPACT ASSESSMENT

Edem Ahiati

Isaac Ato Mensah

The Miller's Impact Assessment Framework is hereby used to show a feasibility assessment of the proposed program (Miller, n.d.). "Every risk must have an owner: orphan risks are not acceptable" (Ketcham & Knight, 2014, p. 16). Therefore we show who will be directly impacted by the respective dimensions of the assisted living program.

DIMENSION	IMPACTS
A. stakeholders directly impacted	Internal stakeholders: Internal stakeholders: 1) King County Council, 2) King County Board of Health, and 3) King County Auditor. The individuals identified in the list of internal stakeholders will more likely feel a direct responsibility to succeed or fail. If the program succeeds, they will more likely feel empowered to continue and improve it. If on the other hand, the town hall meetings fail or there is a lack of consensus about how to proceed, these stakeholders may come under pressure to account for a waste of

resources used in promoting the proposed assisted living program.

External Stakeholders:
External Stakeholders: 1) persons in need of assisted living together with their relatives, 2) community colleges and other training institutions that will train students under the proposed King County Assisted Living Program, 3) integrated delivery systems which already offer assisted living services in Washington State.

These external stakeholders are likely to invest considerable resources into the proposed assisted living program, expecting it to succeed. If all goes well, then they may likely feel they have made a good investment. On the other hand, if the program fails or is discontinued within the foreseeable future, these stakeholders may feel they have wasted their resources in planning and training for such a program.

Elderly persons will more likely become more empowered and more trusting of the government, policymakers and elected officials since they will begin to see that legislation has been made to support assisted living programs. They may also see that the quality of assisted living is improving.

B. anticipated health outcomes	Assisted living in King County will see an improvement. This will show that the King County Government is committed to addressing issues of historical trauma suffered by indigenous peoples (alchemicalmedia, 2013; Harris, 2014).
C. regulatory landscape (e.g., key influencing agencies, regulatory bodies)	The managers of the Medicaid program that provide some funding for the care of the elderly may begin to closely monitor the effectiveness of the King County Assisted Living Program with a view to collaborating with the program staff. This may help the managers of the Medicaid program decide whether or not to commit resources to the assisted living program. The American Association of Retired Persons (AARP) in Seattle and King County may join in the lobbying and advocacy campaigns, if they perceive that the program could benefit their members. The American Association of Retired Persons (AARP) may incur costs for any advocacy programs. This may be a drain on their finances. State agencies often have specific regulations that impact how assisted living facilities are run. State agencies that determine requirements for assisted living facilities and impose penalties may be among the best allies of the King County

	Government since they will usually offer advice on performance standards, and sanction organizations that do not comply with regulations (King County, n.d.).
D. Human resource needs	There is certainly an extra cost to running government services, and the King County Government may begin to feel the impact of resources spent that have made little impact. Organization of health and social care programs will be enhanced positively since health workers will likely perceive that the King County Government is taking more responsibility for assisted living programs. As a result, when there are positive outcomes, there will more likely be a positive impact on employees. It is, therefore, easy to see that all persons on the payroll of the King County Government will put their shoulders to the wheel and see to the creation of the KCALP. During the period of lobbying and advocacy, a considerable number of working hours will be devoted by the King County Government staff to the success of the venture. This can slow down the regular operations of the county if care is not taken because assisted living is a major social issue (Devaney, n.d.; Hatcher, 2020). If, on the other hand, the program succeeds, the King County

	Government may give more resources to the assisted living program office.

MARKET SEGMENTATION

The proposed King County Assisted Living Program (KCALP) builds on the concept of assisted living, either at home or at a care facility and value-based care (Devaney, n.d.; Hatcher, 2020; American Hospital Association, 2014; AARP, 2020). The KCALP also adds to the recently declared holiday to acknowledge the contributions of indigenous people (Kingcountyemployees, 2021). Assisted living programs are already being implemented in the United States, but this program focuses specifically on indigenous people, and deliberately offers them assisted living as a way of combating some of the harmful effects of historical trauma (Devaney, n.d.; Hatcher, 2020; American Hospital Association, 2014; AARP, 2020; alchemicalmedia, 2013; Harris, 2014; Harvard University, n.d.). This program proposes to deliberately target the poorest in America for assistance (County Health Rankings and Roadmap, n.d.). In addition, all poor people who are 65 years and older will benefit when they register for the program. The uniqueness of this proposed program is that it targets indigenous people for sponsored assisted living in their own homes or at caregiving facilities.

15

THE PROSPECTUS FOR THE PROPOSED ASSISTED LIVING PROGRAM FOR KING COUNTY IN WASHINGTON STATE, USA

PART IV: CRITERIA FOR MEASUREMENT

Edem Ahiati

Isaac Ato Mensah

REGULATORY AND LEGAL ENVIRONMENT

The community of elderly persons will become more empowered and more trusting of the government, policymakers and elected officials since they may begin to see that legislation has been passed to support assisted living. It is hereby proposed that the King County Council should pass a vote to approve the expenditure proposed in this business plan which should be financed through mortgage/rental/property tax. That way, anybody who needs assisted living should be supported. King County, as always, implements regulations stipulated by the State of Washington (King County, n.d.). All other guidance such as solid and biomedical waste handling, handling of clients in behavioral health settings, and visitation, insofar as they relate to assisted living facilities must be adhered to by long term care facilities if they are to continue receiving payments from the county for services offered under the King County Assisted Living Program (KCALP) (King County, n.d.). Individual homes must adhere to all regulations, especially on Covid-19 protocols, as determined by the State of Washington, if those homes are to remain registered under the KCALP (King County, n.d.).

HUMAN RESOURCES

There is certainly an extra cost to running government services. The organization of health and social care may be enhanced positively since health workers will begin to see that their government is taking more responsibility for whole-person care and person-centered care. Thus, when there are positive outcomes, there will be a positive impact on employees. It is envisaged that 1000 students will be trained each year for the King County Assisted Living Program. If each training program is offered USD1500 per semester per student for four semesters, that should cost USD6000 per student trained. When this is multiplied by 1000 students, it means King County will spend six million dollars per batch of trainees. The first year of implementation is, therefore, expected to cost six million dollars. If all 1000 people are employed, beginning from the second year, at a gross stipend of USD1000 a month to work on a part-time basis, this will cost one million dollars a month or USD12 million a year in stipends/allowances.

In the second year, therefore, six million dollars spent on training plus 12 million dollars spent on stipends/part-time allowances will add up to 18 million dollars spent on the KCALP from year two onwards. Since the curriculum shall be determined by the community colleges, the training will afford the students the opportunity to seek work elsewhere. Those who opt to work elsewhere shall be required to refund the 6000 dollars spent to support their training. All colleges and large estate owners will be encouraged to donate generously toward the KCALP.

It is envisaged that an office will be created within the King County Government health department to oversee the implementation of the program. The cost of running this office, together with the cost of lobbying and advocacy, and creating and maintaining the proposed register, can easily run into one million dollars. Additional staff may be hired to run this dedicated office and its information technology platforms for the purpose of creating the proposed register. If 10 persons are hired at the cost of USD3,000 a month, that would be USD30,000 a month. In a year that will cost USD360,000. The materials and additional running costs to be spent for smooth operations of the office could cost about USD640,000 a year, thereby bringing the cost of running the proposed King County Assisted Living Program Office to one million dollars. The total cost of training and paying caregivers (USD18 million per annum from the second year); creating the King County Assisted Living Program Office and register (one million dollars per annum); and materials and additional running costs costs (one million dollars per annum) will be USD20 million a year from the second year. In the first year, since there will be no persons to receive the part-time allowances/stipends, the stipends/allowances of USD12 million will not be paid, implying that the first-year cost will be USD8 million.

It is envisaged that 1000 students will be trained and hired each year for the King County Assisted Living Program. Ten new staff will be hired to run the program. These human resources and their attendant expenditure are the main expenditure items. An information technology platform to be designed for the program and its register, and the additional materials and administrative additional running costs are the other cost items envisaged.

CHALLENGES

The Five Whys analysis or Root Cause Analysis designed under the Six-Sigma model will be used for the impact analysis or any circumstances that otherwise may not have been foreseen (Lighter, 2011). The Five Whys model is useful when one wants to go through each identified problem in a step by step manner so that the root cause can be identified and addressed (Lighter, 2011).

This is why it is so simple and effective. By going through each question, one is able to pinpoint the fundamental cause of a problem (Lighter, 2011).

TRACKING SUCCESS

The Kaizen principle will be used to address the challenges posed by the program (Lighter, 2011). Kaizen enables one to measure success in incremental steps, while building on successfully resolved issues or challenges (Lighter, 2011). Adding Kaizen to the Analyze phase of Six Sigma may help reveal additional information (Lighter, 2011). Kaizen is complementary to Six Sigma (Lighter, 2011). It tells us that revolutions in change management are less preferable to an evolutionary process, the latter of which helps organizations to focus on "rapid incremental change" (Lighter, 2011, p. 152). Even if the Five Whys process were exhaustive by any yardstick, during the Analyze phase, by complementing the process with Kaizen, any existing loopholes may be detected (Lighter, 2011).

Kaizen has a time dimension as an important yardstick, which the 5 whys analysis does not have. "As implementation proceeds, the team tracks metrics to determine the need to make rapid corrections to the Kaizen plan (Lighter, 2011, p. 152). Kaizen defines and measures projects into sizable portions "to allow the completion of the intervention within the [one-week] time period" (Lighter, 2011, p. 152). The principle behind Kaizen clearly suggests that the corrective measures that may come through additional questions fundamentally defeat the concept of an exhaustive list of the 5 whys (Lighter, 2011).

Also, the Swiss Cheese Model is a good tool when it comes to analyzing impact and addressing challenges (Lighter, 2011). The Swiss Cheese Model is depicted as several squares of cards, with the tip of each one positioned in the center of the other square, one after the other, in order to expose the other parts of all the squares which may be concealing information that should not go unnoticed (Lighter, 2011). The concealed parts, if not unveiled, may hide information that may render a weak and incomplete analysis. The justification for the Swiss cheese model is that "an error is usually not due to failures with just one system or just one person, but rather shows that multiple systems and processes usually fail to produce an error" (Lighter, 2011, p. 114). This implies that "a one-dimensional review of the failure will miss many of the underlying problems in numerous processes that led to the error" (Lighter, 2011, p. 114).

The success of the assisted living program will be measured by the number of trained caregivers who sign contracts and start working under the King County Assisted Living Program. It will also be measured by assessing the fall rate of persons supported by this program compared to their cohort who are not supported by the program (Acker & Janssen, 2017; Boland et al., 2017; Alvarez et al., 2015; Hatcher, 2020). It will also be measured by the level of satisfaction and happiness expressed by residents and their relatives. It will further be measured by the parameters established by regulatory agencies.

FINANCES

The proposed program will be funded by the taxpayer, and only partly supports the cost of assisted living. It is proposed that the King County Council should pass a vote to approve this spending which will be financed through mortgage/rental/property tax. Elderly people and their relatives will still be conditioned to understand that they must have an abundance mindset and avoid poverty. Besides, a benchmark maximum income level of USD30,000 per annum is required for an individual to qualify - a means-tested approach that will ensure that only about a maximum of about 7% of the adult population in King County will be eligible year-in-year-out (County Health Rankings and Roadmap, n.d.; United States Census Bureau, n.d.). Even so, this 7%, representing about 405,000 people, will not all need assisted living (County Health Rankings and Roadmap, n.d.; United States Census Bureau, n.d.). Throughout the U.S, about 730,000 people live in assisted living facilities, implying that King County which is a subset of the U.S., will have fewer numbers to deal with (Neufeld, 2017).

King County has a population of about 2.2 million people with 13 percent of them being 65 years and older, implying that the uppermost limit of eligible people will be 286,000 (AARP, 2020). However, not all these people are poor or need help with assisted living. This analysis ensures that the program targets a specific population so that the financing of the program will become sustainable over the foreseeable future.

REVENUE

If each training program is offered USD1,500 per student per semester for four semesters of training, that should cost USD6,000 per student trained over two years. When this is multiplied by 1000 students, it means King County will spend six million dollars a year training these students. The first year of implementation (two semesters) is, therefore, expected to cost three million dollars. If all 1,000 people are employed beginning from the second year, at a gross stipend of USD1,000 a month to work on a part-time basis, this will cost one million dollars a month, or USD12 million a year in stipends/allowances.

In the second year, therefore, six million dollars spent on the training program annually plus 12 million dollars spent on stipends/part-time allowances will add up to at least 18 million dollars spent on the Assisted Living Program from year two onwards. Since the curriculum shall be determined by the community colleges, the training will afford those who successfully complete the program and get certified the opportunity to seek work elsewhere. Those who opt to work elsewhere shall be required to refund the USD6000 spent in supporting their training. It is envisaged that an office will be created within the King County Government offices to oversee the implementation of the program. The cost of running this office, together with the cost of lobbying and advocacy, and creating and maintaining the proposed register, can easily run into one million dollars.

Additional staff will be hired to run this dedicated office and its information technology platforms. If 10 persons are hired at the cost of US$3,000 a month, that would be USD30,000 a month. The salaries for the 10 additional personnel will, therefore, cost USD360,000 per annum. The materials and additional running costs to be spent for smooth operations of the office could cost about US$640,000 a year, thereby bringing the cost of running the proposed King County Assisted Living Program Office to one million dollars per year.

The total cost of training and paying caregivers (US$18 million per annum from the second year); creating the King County Assisted Living Program Office and register (one million dollars per annum); and materials, labor and additional running costs (one million dollars per annum) will be USD20 million a year from the second year. In the first year, since there will be no persons to receive the part-time allowances/stipends, the stipends/allowances estimated at US\$12 million per annum will not be paid, implying that the first-year cost will be USD8 million. This means that the expenditure of the King County Government will go up, with the introduction of this new additional expenditure item.

FINANCIAL RISKS

It is envisaged that from year three onwards, an additional average expenditure of US\$12 million will be added to the county's budget. This money will be used to pay trained and licensed caregivers. Since the baby boom generation is growing older, many more people are joining the community of old persons, and the problem of nursing homes is a serious national problem, these annual increments should be expected and absorbed by the King County Government as a necessary intervention to ensure quality assisted living (AARP, 2020; Khimm, 2021).

IMPACT ON HEALTH OUTCOMES

If the number of falls among persons 65 years and older reduces significantly as a result of increased penetration of assisted living programs, that will be an indicator of success (Acker & Janssen, 2017; Boland et al., 2017; Alvarez et al., 2015; Hatcher, 2020; Bu et al., 2020). By comparison, persons under assisted living programs are expected to experience less falls than those who live alone if the right care is given following evidence-based best practice approaches to caregiving (Acker & Janssen, 2017; Boland et al., 2017; Alvarez et al., 2015; Hatcher, 2020; Bu et al., 2020).

Elderly people who suffer falls at home are a serious health problem. The proposed King County Assisted Living Program will, therefore, help to minimize that risk (Acker & Janssen, 2017; Boland et al., 2017; Alvarez et al., 2015; Hatcher, 2020). This prospectus supports a mixture of either home-based assisted living or institution-based assisted living, depending on client preferences. This is based on the outcome of solid research that suggests that "the impact of home care compared to alternative care locations on [...] health outcomes [of the elderly] is heterogeneous" (Boland et al., 2017, para. 4).

16

BUILDING THE CASE OF THE FOUR MOST RURAL REGIONS OF GHANA

Isaac Ato Mensah

The average life expectancy at birth for Ghana is 66.3 years as of 2019, compared to the global average of 73.3 years (World Health Organization, n.d.). This figure is an increase by 6.5 years from 2000 to 2019, a period of 19 years. This means in 2000, the average life expectancy for persons living in Ghana was 59.78 years. There are similar numbers for many developing countries. We all must, therefore, take this Gray Matter as our personal battle in our respective families, districts, county's boroughs, boulevards and provinces. With perseverance and fortitude exhibited over time, a passionate District Chief Executive (DCE), governor, senator, or council president may heed the global call to action and declare assisted living for the aged a security threat. Then the DCE, governor, council chair - whatever the honorable designation is - given their mandate as chairperson of the district/county/borough/provincial/boulevard/street security committee will marshall all state agencies under their command to achieve this task.

A Rutgers University professor of anthropology, after at least eight years of research on care of the aged in southern Ghana has confirmed the power of the Ghanaian family in caring for the aged (Coe, 2021). However, there is no serious policy direction for state institutions to provide assisted living or safeguarding for the aged (Coe, 2021). Coe (2021) rightly observed that there are various promising private schemes toward care for the aged, but they remain unaffordable to most families. It is with this backdrop that we advocate that district assemblies must guarantee care for the aged. After all, they are mandated by law to coordinate all state agencies under their care to achieve this all important mandate. A nation - make it a district - that does not honor its senior citizens is not worth dying for.

In the case of Ghana, unlike Coe (2021), we prefer the district assemblies to coordinate this task, firstly, by enlisting families. When the district assemblies have the numbers, then they can rope in other state agencies because the assemblies can get wide consultation and collaboration across the board. From our experience as practitioners/decision makers/employees/participant observers, the Ghana Health Service (GHS) as suggested by Coe (2021) is not fit for purpose, for several reasons.

One, the GHS is preoccupied with institutional care or if you will the First Curve of health care which involves getting patients to come to hospital. Two, in their planning, the GHS will in all likelihood seek budgetary support from the central government and the so-called Development Partners such as international non-governmental organisations. This bureaucratic process will make this all important task remain forever on the drawing board. Three, the GHS does not have administrative control over private hospitals even though the former often pretends to have such powers. Therefore, the suggestion by Coe (2021) that the GHS should be the coordinating agency since they manage community health nurses assigned to local clinics will be ineffective. The community health nurses are employed by GHS. Coe (2021) continued, "It would seem simple and easy to expand the mission of the community health nurses beyond maternal and child health, to include the care of older adults" (para. 19). Professor Coe's important seminal work failed to look at health sector data, for example, the Second Curve concepts that strongly suggest the need for dedicated teams for value-based care (American Hospital Association, 2014).

Given the limitations of the GHS, they are unable to solicit the fullest cooperation with non-governmental healthcare agencies within the respective districts in which they operate. In the districts of Ghana, the GHS operates as the District Health Management Team (DHMT). Even among the government established healthcare agencies, it is almost anathema for the GHS to attempt getting compliance from the Teaching hospitals, for example, because they, the teaching hospitals, are independent agencies under Ghana's Ministry of Health. For this reason, any policy implementation undertaken by the DHMTs on behalf of the Ministry of Health will in all likelihood yield suboptimal results.

The district assemblies in Ghana, on the other hand, are relatively smaller institutions with elected and non-elected assembly members. They generate enough revenue and are mandated by law to promote the development of their districts. They have the power to coordinate all state agencies within their respective jurisdictions. They can raise taxes. They can also use coercive, incentive and combination policies to achieve their objectives (Cao & Chen, 2018; Lai, 2022; McCoy, 2019). We, therefore, respectfully disagree with the renowned anthropologist when she says "community health nurses" should be given "some basic geriatric training to help individuals and households manage chronic conditions like falls, stroke, diabetes, hypertension, and dementia" (Coe, 2021, para. 20). Safeguarding the aged is serious business everywhere in the developed world.

Hence, the developing world cannot have it any other way. Ghana and the rest of the developing world, for that matter, need training and recruiting agencies licensed by the respective district assemblies. When these agencies and their employees mess up they could get sued or face sanctions such as withdrawal of their licenses. Yes, we mean both the agencies and their carers/caregivers should obtain separate district assembly licenses to operate an agency and practice caregiving respectively.

This critique is in no way an attempt to take away an iota of credit from the all important seminal work that Professor Coe has done in Ghana. Coe's work is an important exploratory study that forms the basis for understanding the Gray Matter of nursing care homes in Ghana. In scholarship, we cannot proceed without identifying the foundation works of earlier researchers, hence this critique. However, there are important perspectives that must be brought to bear on the matter, just as our work is also subject to critique by other reviewers.

Now to the data that justifies assisted living program in Ghana. According to the Ghana Statistical Service (2021), the Western North, Savannah, Upper East and Upper West Regions have the most rural populations with a share of 70.2%, 70.4%, 73.6% and 74.6% respectively compared to their respective urban populations. This means that only 30% of people in each of these respective regions live in the urban parts of the regions. We, therefore, suggest these four regions as the model regions for experimenting with/piloting a home based and nursing care home program. It is clear that these four regions have more rural people per capita than the rest of Ghana. They also, of course, have more rural areas, hence lack more social amenities including hospitals and the best trained healthcare workers. The historical disadvantages they have suffered have implications for historical trauma. Thus any health rescue mission should not fail to consider these four regions. Upper East Region has a population density of 28.8 thereby placing it in the top five for Ghana and close to the national average of 25.9. Western North (16.8), Upper West (10.3) and Savannah (5.3) are in the bottom seven and more sparsely dispersed than the national average. This further evidence corroborates the evidence on the ground that these selected regions have suboptimal healthcare facilities. The best they can hope for is the so-called Community Health and Planning Services (CHPS) compounds, staffed by Community Nurses and other healthcare workers who cannot diagnose nor prescribe any medications.

Yet another indicator is the national average household size for Ghana. This was 3.6 in 2021, but 4.5 in 2010. For Savannah the figure was 7.1 in 2010 but reduced to 4.9 in 2021 (change; -2.2) which is indicative of rural-urban migration. For the Upper East Region the figure declined from 5.9 to 4.8, (change; -1.8) still lower than the 2021 average national household size of 3.6. Upper West Region also improved from 6.4 to 4.6, (change; -1.1) still lower than the national average. Western North Region meanwhile decreased from 4.6 to 3.6, (change; -0.9) aligning exactly with the national average (Ghana Statistical Service, 2021). While it may appear a good thing for the numbers to be shrinking, it is also a further indication that more of the youthful population who usually stay in the rural areas and take care of the elderly are migrating to the urban areas to find jobs and other sources of livelihood.

If such youth send home remittances, that is a positive outcome, but who remains to take care of the elderly now becomes a growing national crisis. Now to more grim data. Western North Region has a population of 880,921 (male, 451,948; female, 428,973) (Ghana Statistical Service, 2021). The non-household population here is 11,165 (male, 5,116; female, 6,049). Where these people sleep could be in front of shops or at the lorry stations. This is where the population health interventions must map out these people and target the aged among them for assisted living services. Savannah Region has an estimated 2021 population of 653,266 (male, 327,687; female, 325,579). This comprises 6,485 persons who have no households to live in (male, 3,369; female, 3,116). The population recorded for the Upper East Region was 1,301,226 (male, 631,263; female, 669,963). Those in non-households are 29,154 (male, 14,123; female, 15,031).

Last but not least, the population captured for the Upper West Region was 901,502 (male, 440,317; female, 461,185). Among the non-household dwellers of 26,028, males were 13,014 while females were the same 13,014 (Ghana Statistical Service, 2021). These are regional figures, hence on a district basis, it should be far easier to locate these persons and map out the elderly among them for intervention.

Now that Ghana is rolling out a national identification card system, identifying persons by age for population health assistance, especially with assisted living should not pose much of a challenge. Indeed on a district basis, in the Western North Region, the non-household residents range from a high of 2,956 (the highest being females at 1704) persons in Sefwi Wiawso Municipality to the lowest 108 (the lowest being males; 44) persons in Bodi district. On a rural basis, the figures range from a high of 1,483 (highest being females; 997) persons in Sefwi Bibiani Anhwiaso Bekwai district to the lowest of 2 (the lowest being females at zero) persons in

Suaman district (Ghana Statistical Service, 2021). Mapping out the elderly aged sixty and above on a district by district basis should, therefore, be a fairly routine task for well-trained government workers collaborating with each other across state institutions. Ditto for Upper West, Upper East and Savannah Regions.

In the case of Ghana, the Directive Principles of State Policy enjoin the state and its agencies to avoid discrimination on the basis of age, sex, ethnicity, language, etc. Specifically, Article 35(2) of the Ghana's Constitution states: "The President shall report to Parliament at least once a year all the steps taken to ensure the realization of the policy objectives contained in this Chapter; and in particular, the realization of basic human rights, a healthy economy, the right to work, the right to good health care and the right to education".

Again, according to article 35(3) of the Constitution, "The State shall provide just and reasonable access by all citizens to public facilities and services in accordance with law". The Ghanaian Constitution is even more generous/forward looking in using the term safeguard in article 35(2) thus: "The State shall protect and safeguard…..and shall seek the wellbeing of all her citizens". We submit humbly, therefore, that the aged in our rural areas and throughout Ghana do not have that fair and just access to healthcare.

Even if it is argued that the whole nation is marching gradually towards a more just and reasonable access, the aged, with all the historical trauma they have endured should have priority access, as an affirmative action and in solidarity with the fact that we all are desirous of becoming senior citizens. This is provided for in Article 35(5) of the Ghanaian constitution which says that the state shall prohibit discrimination and prejudice on the grounds of circumstances of birth, among other grounds. As such, District Assemblies must sit up and perform their obligations of providing quality health and education for their aged populace.

Several financing models could be considered. One, there could be a coercive policy by District Assembly bye-laws to compel the working population to take care of their aged parents.

However, coercive policies could backfire when the breadwinners of the family lose their jobs. Besides, it is already customary in Ghana for breadwinners to take care of their aged dependents. Therefore, why not a combination policy involving coercion (that is, for example, a bye-law that requires homeowners/tenants to hire a caregiver for their aged relatives) and incentives (that is, tax breaks, awards/promotions for organizations that fund caregivers and their training institutions)? The beautiful thing about this policy is that the District Assemblies will register the training agencies that register the caregivers. This could be a source of jobs and revenues. Governmental policy instruments could be either coercive policies, incentive policies, and combination policies (Cao & Chen, 2018; Lai, 2022; McCoy, 2019).

Bali et al. (2021) observed that there could be several combinations of the three. For instance, the Government of Ghana promotes safe driving campaigns during the Christmas and Easter seasons - a period when alcoholism rises and contributes to road traffic accidents. At the same time, the government punishes speeding drivers.

Ghanaians in the diaspora, especially, who have been looking forward to some high standards and regulation will also have the assurance that only trained/licensed personnel will handle their aged relatives. Assisted living programs will now, hopefully, become an integral part of many academic courses even beyond Nursing because it could offer employment opportunities for those who may want to look wider for more employment opportunities. Medical Doctors will have the assurance that the aged will be assisted at home to follow through with their respective treatment plans. Co-financing models could also be envisaged in which case, the aged person's relatives may pay a part of the labor cost. In short, everybody will be the winner.

17

JUSTIFICATION FOR THE PROPOSED DISTRICT ASSEMBLIES ASSISTED LIVING PROGRAM

Isaac Ato Mensah

On a visit to Pori, Finland in 2014, I took up the issue of old age care with Mr B, an acquaintance. Starting a family early while lacking the means to take care of them optimally versus planning to start late when you have acquired some property versus when you choose to not start a family of your own is a crucial Gray Matter that everyone must reckon with. "In Ghana, children are our social security," I remarked rather blandly, as we reflected on life. In many wealthy countries such as Finland, Sweden, The Netherlands, Lithuania and Japan, many people have no need to worry about giving birth. The social security that comes from giving birth and expecting grown up children to return the favor of taking care of aged parents is provided for in a government regulated welfare system. Hence, neither Mr. B nor his parents were expecting him to do any such chores of forking out cash and assisting with activities of daily living. Besides, both parents were earning good monthly pension remittances. Furthermore, "the government takes care of them in the old people's home when assisted living is required," Mr B proudly affirmed. "The oldies look forward to spending good time in those residential nursing care homes with their fellow senior citizens. They play a lot of games. They are given very nutritious food. They just love the community and they are happier there." I asked why anyone would leave their biological family and stay away forever with a new set of people until death do them part. "Staying at home will rather make them lonely because your grown up children will have to go to work so they cannot visit you as often as you may want," my acquaintance supplied.

It all made sense now. But is happiness subjective; just an attitude of the mind; or there can be an objective criteria for measuring happiness? Regardless, there is a World Happiness Report - compiled since 2002 - which consistently ranks the Finnish among some of the happiest people on earth. Assisted living in Finland, a nation with universal health insurance is certainly a good example for Ghana and many other low and middle income countries with no universal health insurance coverage. The Scandinavian countries such as Finland, Sweden, Denmark, Iceland and Norway - in no particular order - usually perform consistently better due partly to their welfare programs which the aged generally benefit from. They are also among the happiest people in the world, with Finland taking the number one position both in 2020 and 2021, the two most recent years for which data is available (World Population Review, n.d.).

Perhaps the longest study on human happiness, undertaken by Harvard University for at least 75 years involving over 750 persons, established this conclusion: "Good relationships keep us happier and healthier" (Waldinger, 2015). The closest the Ministry of Health (MOH) of the Republic of Ghana has come to doing anything about safeguarding the aged is in the area of a national healthcare Quality Assurance (QA) proposal. After four years, the Quality Assurance draft documents were abandoned without implementation. As of the time of publishing this book, there was a new Quality Assurance proposal on the table. Ghana's MOH has been licensing nursing homes for the aged in recent years through its Health Facilities Regulatory Agency (HeFRA).

We must point out that often in Ghana, civil/public servants can frustrate serious minded parties that want to establish a world-class organization. They may use red tape bureaucracy to frustrate your investments. If you are reading this and you intend to assist some aged persons in Ghana foot their bill for a nursing home, to establish one yourself, offer collaboration services for nursing homes, or pursue the need for full disclosure of public information, please do not give up. Our experience is that civil/public servants often resort to stonewalling when their official records are not updated and/or there are some shenanigans going on. For example, employees could dread the consequences of providing the list of registered nursing homes. This is because of the dread of later withdrawing some nursing home licenses because some vigilant parties took on the HeFRA in the overall public interest.

It is instructive to note that the National Aging Policy on Ghana proposes an Active Aging Fund. Let us take a peep into it: "Government will contribute the seed money for the fund and each year the MMDAs [Metropolitan, Municipal and District Assemblies] will contribute a specific percentage of the District Assembly Common Fund (DACF) as their contribution to the Active Ageing Fund in their districts. The private sector employers, NGOs [Non-Governmental Organizations], development partners [foreign donors] and philanthropists will be encouraged to contribute to the Active Ageing Fund" (National Aging Policy: 'Ageing with Security and Dignity', 2010, p. 65). OK, everyone, that was 2010, 13 years ago. Yeah, right; the government of Ghana is looking forward to yet another talkshop at a hotel near you where the donors can give them some doughnuts.

But we digress. This is all the more reason we all should remain focused on our elderly folk and what you and your District Assembly can do for them. No need to rely on the central government. Let us handle this Gray Matter on the familial level first. Then at the community level. Thence to the District Assembly or local council or county or provincial level, whichever nomenclature is applicable in your country. Given our Ghanaian experience, we do not advocate for central government planning in our suggestions.

Now to a familial level experience of caregiving/safeguarding. In the 1990s a model hospital for total nursing care was built in Cape Coast Ghana, named the Cape Coast Teaching Hospital. The indigenous folk have christened the hospital Interberton, the name of the contractors. Interbeton is a model hospital for nurses.

When my grand aunty Sophia Williams, then a septuagenarian, was admitted at Interberton circa 2010, my siblings and I traveled all the way from Accra with food for our beloved Aunty Sophia because it would have been frankly uncustomary not to do so.

I was a practicing Health Services Administrator at the time, and I admired the firmness and professionalism with which the nurses politely declined our request to deliver home cooked food to the patient. In the end the nurses accepted the food, but without mincing words with us that they would put it down and decide at a conference whether or not to serve it to the patient. The nurses were proud to promote total nursing care. There were many other patient relatives who were going through similar negotiations to deliver bread, assorted fruits, soups and other foods. My cousin Ekua Gloria was allowed in there as the only relative to support in giving bed baths, after a hard-fought negotiation. Even then Ekua told us that the nurses always did the bed bath themselves, always insisting proudly that it was their duty.

In Ghana if you do not take care of your sick relatives, you will incur direct insults from your neighbors. And rumors about your lack of proper home training will spread like bushfire. But how did Aunty Sophia end up in hospital? She stood on a low kitchen stool to compensate for her height disadvantage and tried hanging clothes on a drying line at home in Elmina. Unfortunately, she fell down and broke her hip because apparently the stool became slippery with water! Hitherto, she had never needed assistance with activities of daily living. This was a routine she had done all the time. She always believed - as many seniors her age do - that performing her own daily tasks would make her stay fit. The caregiving at home and hospital by Ekua Gloria, the granddaughter, was exceptional; Ekua had been properly trained by the old lady for such a role as many Ghanaian women are trained to do. But the full time job took all of Ekua Gloria's time. She spent at least two years on the caregiving job post surgery and her stress was obvious. Full time. Under our proposed District Assemblies Assisted Living Program (DAALP) extensively discussed in this book, home-trained carers/caregivers such as Ekua Gloria can receive formal training, certification and salaries/allowances for their services. The Ghanaian resort to home-trained caregivers is not entirely different from that of the Philippines where due to lack of optimal institutional care by the government, family members are trained to care for the aged at home (Badana & Andel, 2018).

Caregivers go through a lot of stress as the empirical evidence from several studies shows (Lozano et al., 2020; Liu et al., 2020; Sherman, 2019). In Ghana it is not uncommon to have patients' relatives work side by side with nurses, ward assistants and orderlies in a hospital setting. The negative effect of patient relatives working as caregivers is that they are the veritable conduit through whom alternative medicines enter the wards. Such medications are usually hidden away from the nursing team in the bags and cabinets of the patients. It should not be too far-fetched to imagine that as nursing care homes multiply in Ghana, relatives who are caregivers will carry over this practice from the hospital environment into the residential and nursing care homes. Beyond that, patient relatives who work as caregivers have reported a lot of stress.

Lozano et al. (2020) did a systematic review of 27 studies done in 11 countries. These combined studies involved 689 caregivers. Lozano et al. (2020) concluded that poor mental health and well-being is often the plight of caregivers. The caregivers also faced barriers to practicing their tasks, obviously from health workers. Indeed, if family carers are not moderated they will likely suffer cognitive, emotional and physical breakdown in the long run (Sherman, 2019).

But family caregivers in Ghana will not give up; they deem it their obligation, their safeguarding duty, to invigilate poorly paid and lowly motivated healthcare workers in an increasingly dysfunctional healthcare system. Is that not the necessary pushback to be expected in the face of failed states and failing state institutions? All told, a ready-and-willing pool of family volunteers abound who could be trained for caregiving and safeguarding duties.

Under the proposed District Assemblies Assisted Living Program (DAALP), eligible senior citizens who register will receive financial or human resource support for assisted living. These human resources are already motivated, direct relatives who will receive training and obtain professional licenses from registered care agencies as already indicated in this book. This will show a shift from volume-based care to value-based care (County Health Rankings and Roadmap, n.d.).

This solution, the proposed DAALP, promotes value-based care such that no persons who need assisted living will be left behind (American Hospital Association, 2014). You could also name the concept County Assisted Living Program (CALP) or Provincial Assisted Living Program (PALP).

This proposed assisted living program offers more efficiency in caregiving since the subscribers can either stay at home or receive care through an assisted living facility. More likely, the clients/subscribers who are the direct oldies in need of assisted living will not feel emotionally separated from their loved ones when they are at home receiving the needed care. Those who may opt to go to long term care facilities may, however, feel emotionally separated when they go into a care facility under the DAALP.

UNIQUE SELLING PROPOSITION

The District Assembly Assisted Living Program (DAALP) will promote assisted living, which is an essential part of value-based care (American Hospital Association, 2014). This will show that the district assemblies are committed to addressing the problems created by historical trauma, especially trauma suffered by indigenous peoples (Harris, 2014; Harvard University, n.d.; alchemicalmedia, 2013).

Aged people who experience falls at home are a serious health problem (AARP, 2020; Hatcher, 2020; Bu et al., 2020). The proposed DAALP will, therefore, help to minimize that risk. This proposal supports a mixture of home-based assisted living or institution-based assisted living, depending on client/subscriber preferences. This is based on the research evidence that there is a "heterogeneous" health outcome between falls for residents versus those cared for at home (Boland et al., 2017, para. 4). Findings comparing home care to institutional care were mixed. As indicated elsewhere in this book, most reviews found no differences in health outcomes between rehabilitation at home versus conventional rehabilitation services" (Boland et al., 2017, para. 3).

18

THE SECRET OF PRAYER

Isaac Ato Mensah

"We enter onto the broad road of perdition when we neglect prayer" - Saint Paul of the Cross

Many people are religious/spiritual. That itself is a source of faith, strength and hope that they will get better. This faith helps the medical team to accomplish their treatment goals in collaboration with the resident and their relatives. Therefore, it is important that caregivers support residents to maintain a healthy spiritual life. At least the religious/spiritual life they routinely practiced prior to enrolling in an assisted living program should not be compromised.

According to Pope John Paul II, "Faith and reason are like two wings on which the human spirit rises to the contemplation of truth; and God has placed in the human heart a desire to know the truth—in a word, to know himself—so that, by knowing and loving God, men and women may also come to the fullness of truth about themselves" (Crossroads Initiative, n.d., para. 2). This presents a challenge for caregivers in how they allow the two worlds of faith and reason or science to flourish side by side in a care home, since they are not mutually exclusive.

It is not unexpected to find many healthcare facilities in Ghana inundated with letters from religious groups that want to offer prayers and or make donations. All staff should be properly oriented with a welcoming attitude to such groups. At the same time, the management should be firm in vetting any such groups and the content of their messages. In a developing country context, many of the religious groups are run by persons with suboptimal training especially in guidance and counseling, and clinical psychology. This could pose serious problems as religious fundamentalism abounds within such groups. Worse still, the TV stations are flooded with movies that attribute almost every human problem to some human beings who are pulling some strings in the spiritual realm. The mind control game that goes on in these parts of the world is simply outrageous. The Kingdom of Morocco, for example, offers training in moderate Islam to Imams from La Côte D'Ivoire (North African Post, 2016). This helps to promote religious tolerance since the training offers a veritable and progressive worldview against radicalisation. Pope John Paull II urged that theologians should interpret science with philosophical lenses (Russell, n.d.). This he hoped would reduce the gap between seekers after truth via human experience/history and those who look to nature to discover their own truths (Russell, n.d.).

The mystery about death is that it is part of life (Mensah, 2019b). One of the best places to experience this reality is in a healthcare center. In such an environment, you become more humbled by the reality of your daily existence. You know without reading, without anyone, nor any textbook reinforcing it, that as a health worker, you only offer treatment, and God heals the disease, a position clearly elucidated by Dr NAB Andrews, Chief of Neurosurgery and Vice President of neuroGhana through my various interactions with him. Westerners do not often wear their religion on their sleeve like the way many people in West Africa. In many parts of the world, some patients may sometimes arrange for priests to give them Holy Communion and or blessings at a hospice or nursing care home. Some persons are able to arrange for their aged residents to attend exclusive weekly church services near the hospital/nursing home/hospice, usually midweek. In many parts of the world, some churches organize Christmas, Easter or holiday church services, or parties for the aged. The hospitals usually have chaplains. This makes it easier to find a priest/Imam. Many people request for a priest or their equivalent in other religions to minister to the religious/spiritual needs of the residents.

19

WHY YOU NEED AN INDIVIDUAL END OF LIFE CARE PLAN NOW

Florence Afful

Isaac Ato Mensah

How many people do you want at your funeral? Shocking question? Then fasten your seatbelt. We're going to take you right through difficult terrain. But it's for your own good. We just want you to peep into the realities of a nursing care home so that you can best advise yourself.

An end of life care plan, also known as an advance care plan (ACP) is a necessary evil to keep each and everyone of us from embarrassing death and funeral arrangements (National Institute for Health and Care Excellence, n.d.). You know you will die one day, don't you? Do you already foresee that your extended family will fight over your corpse as often happens in some parts of the world? Do you think your young children will be able to decide with the medical team whether or not to continue your hospital treatment? Who will organize your funeral? You're getting the drift, aren't you?

Let's get down to more horrid situations. Now fancy some hired neighborhood young men dancing with your coffin as they carry your mortal remains to the cemetery! And they're throwing your dead body out of the coffin mistakenly onto the streets! Such horrendous situations have happened in Ghana on a few occasions with videos of such mishaps going viral. Are you convinced already that you must plan your end of life care plan/advance care plan now?

An end of life care plan is prepared when the person is able to discuss, communicate and consent to a care plan with a medical team (Akdeniz et al., 2021). In other words, the ideal situation is now - when an adult is able to make a decision without any mental incapacitation or force whatsoever. The next best situation is when you cannot decide and the person who has authority over your care, say, your next of kin is consulted over your end of life care plan (Akdeniz et al., 2021). That's when we put this care plan in place.

When we get someone who is able to understand the information, even in the presence of the family, we ask them: what do you want; your best wishes? Maybe some persons will say: "I want to die peacefully in my sleep in a nursing home". Or: "I want to be resuscitated". Or: "I want to be sent to a hospital to die". Or: "I want my family to be close to me and around me during my last hours of death". Those that opt to not be resuscitated usually do so when there is no quality of life. For example, when they are in a vegetative state. "In such a case, why do I want to be resuscitated?", one may say. "For what?" Such persons understand philosophically that there is no quality of life. With those that are able to walk around or do some stuff at old age, the relatives do not usually consent to: "DO NOT RESUSCITATE," so really, it depends on the state of the case (Akdeniz et al., 2021). Sometimes also the person is able to decide but they may say: "Oh no, I don't want to be resuscitated if such an occasion arises". The resident's family may then agree with them that they should not be resuscitated. Should we find the person gasping or dying we should let the person die peacefully, they may suggest. Some are very old but able to walk, or hold onto the bars in the corridor and walk. Some are able to walk with Zimmer frames. All these examples mean that it depends on the choices or wishes of the residents and their respective families.

Other responses could be: "I want to be cremated". Still others: "I want to be buried". All these scenarios boil down to one of two options: 1) does the resident have the mental capacity to understand and decide on what is being said, or 2) if not then the family must take the decision for the person.

If the person has insurance plans in place we get all such information and write their care plan. Whether the person wants cremation, or whether the person wants to be buried is particularly noted. Where there is nothing like that, sometimes the relatives may indicate that when that time comes the staff should call them and they will arrange at that time. Clearly, every family is different, depending on whether they have money and have bought the insurance already, or when the person dies then they do that arrangement. These end of life decisions make things easy for everyone.

It is not an easy discussion to have; to meet a family and ask them about the death wishes of their relatives. It's really a difficult kind of meeting to do. Yet it has to be done so that at the end it will not be so stressful (Schulz & Sherwood, 2008). Your relative is dying and you're now having to arrange this and that?! In short, that's the benefit of having an end of life care plan. If you're able to put that in place, then, when that difficult time comes you won't have the extra stress of going through these unavoidable conversations. It also saves time and makes the burial quick. Needless to say, delayed burials have financial implications. Besides, the person's wishes are fulfilled; not somebody else's wishes.

In Ghana, for example, when somebody dies, there are first meetings, second meetings, family going to meet to discuss the burial permit, et cetera, et cetera. Our experience in Ghana is that when you try to have such conversations with family members, their usual response is that either you want them to die or you are wishing to die. But no, it's your wish; what your soul wants. Even the songs you want played you are able to say during such conversations. Do you want a horse ride with your hearse? A limousine ride with a chauffeur? Then there is the funeral service, if you so desire. The priest to preach the sermon/homily at your funeral service. What the priest should preach about. Whatever you wish. The flowers and all. The graveside. The songs. You can choose the songs that you like. Everything will be done according to your wishes.

As glamorous as it sounds, as we have indicated here, these are no easy conversations (Schulz & Sherwood, 2008). It's a difficult decision to make, so sometimes we cannot have advance wishes in place. Some persons make the decision at the last minute. Still, when they do we should keep all that information and have it in place for those who will implement the wishes.

What are the medications that are likely to be given at the end of life stage? Life could sometimes become hard. We all know that. But when a dying person is in pain they need to be managed so that they become pain-free. Thus will they die peacefully without being in pain. Do you agree or disagree? When residents are assessed, depending on the condition, some of them are put on Control Drugs (CD Drugs) also known as CD medication. For pain relief, they could be prescribed morphine, oxycodone, Butrans Patch (Buprenorphine) and other similar medication (Anekar et al., 2023; BMA, 2017). Midazolam is particularly recommended when the resident is agitated so that it can relax them (Mayo Clinic, n.d.).

There is also glycopyrronium (Glycopyrrolate). This is used when the respiratory tract and especially the tongue get relaxed such that there is too much secretion. This medication is then prescribed to control the secretions (Gallanosa et al., 2023). This may be given as injections or oral medications. Some persons, especially those in hospices, may be prescribed strong analgesics that are inserted into the subcutaneous (under the skin), via a procedure called syringe drive. The syringe drive is done every 10 minutes, 20 minutes or 30 minutes, depending on the severity of the pain. Others are on a syringe drive every single hour! Twenty-four hours a day! Every day of the week! Phew! In other words, chronic pain is a daily existential reality for some people. Until they depart this mortal life! Such persons need our empathy, sympathy, support, love and care - on a daily basis. "The [International Association for the Study of Pain] IASP defines chronic pain as pain that has persisted beyond normal tissue healing time" (BMA, 2017, p. 3). Felman (2023) affirms that it is difficult to get an objective criteria for diagnosing pain.

Therefore, it is what you tell the Medical Doctor that will be used to make a diagnosis and subsequently determine a treatment plan (Felman, 2023). In a nursing care home the nurses/carers may also use their intuition and experience/expertise to prepare a report about your medical history. This will help the Medical Doctors to review your pain medication. Felman (2023) references a 2016 study about biased perceptions against people with ethnic African antecedents that they have thicker skin, hence feel less pain. The use of intuition and expertise to understand and decipher the pain that the patient/resident is going through thus becomes even more complicated. But why does pain occur? It's due to tissue damage which has been communicated to the brain via the spinal cord. As in the case of chronic pain, as per the definition by the British Medical Association earlier referenced, the tissue is not healing as expected (BMA, 2017).

St Christopher's is an example of a hospice that provides palliative care under regulation by the Quality Care Commission of the UK (St Christopher's, n.d.). In conditions whereby a decision has been made that no more treatment is needed because it will not make any difference, residents may be referred to a hospice. An example of such a condition is cancer. Needless to say, chronic pain is a critical Gray Matter that must be discussed at some point in time when cancer is being treated.

During the end of life stage of a person, they may be discharged from a hospital to a nursing care home with the expectation that they are going to die in a few weeks or months. But they may stay alive for even two years, thus defying expectations. Others die earlier than expected.

Finally, we must distinguish between a residential care home and a nursing care home. Residential care homes are usually staffed by Carers with virtually no professional Nurses on duty. Nurses may come around, say, weekly, monthly or at such intervals depending on a resident's need. Residential care homes are recommended for persons who are able to do their own daily routine; they only need minimal assistance with assisted daily living; and have the (mental) capacity to make decisions as well. Nursing care homes, on the other hand, are recommended for such residents when their ability to undertake routine tasks become problematic (Neufeld, 2017).

SUMMARY AND CONCLUSION

Isaac Ato Mensah

Florence Afful

To summarize our case for safeguarding the aged as a global population health crisis, we show the linkages between loss of indigenous languages, as an example, and its association with historical trauma and Alzheimer's Disease (AD). AD is one of the many conditions that nursing homes, professional Nurses and Caregivers have to contend with on a daily basis. We then further buttress our argument by presenting you with the population pyramids of some of the countries with the best healthcare systems, compared to those with some of the worst. This is to enable you to equally draw your own conclusions on the matter. Thence follows the conclusion which simply says that safeguarding the aged will make them - and us all - happy and joyous. Hence, all humankind should put their shoulders to the wheel.

SUMMARY

Item 1.3 of the Sustainable Development Goals (SDGs) states: "Implement nationally appropriate social protection systems and measures for all, including floors, and by 2030 achieve substantial coverage of the poor and the vulnerable" (The Danish Institute for Human Rights, n.d.). This target rightly considers the cultural context of the environment within which assisted living and/or nursing care home strategies are to be implemented. As we have demonstrated throughout this book, various indigenous peoples have suffered historical trauma including being forced to abandon their language. They have thereby lost significant portions of their cultural wealth/capital which has made them poorer. Since those indigenous peoples are offering the necessary push back, any behavior change communication targeted at them will not be effective unless there is an intervention. "In reality, the marginalization and demise of minority languages leads to destruction of intellectual and philosophical concepts and perspectives; it should be resisted in democratic and progressive societies by all enlightened people" (Mensah, 2019a, para. 24). Thus, the United Nations devoted considerable time and resources to celebrate the International Year of Indigenous Languages (IYIL 2019) (Mensah, 2019a). "Language impairments are usually one of the first cognitive signs of the onset of AD [Alzheimer's Disease]. Specifically, they are caused by a decrease of sociolinguistic aspects. These include the meaning of words, difficulties with finding a relevant word, naming, and word comprehension" (Kilmova et al, 2015, para. 12). Otherwise, you may try a worthy intervention at safeguarding, but culture will eat strategy for lunch (Becker's Hospital Review, n.d.). Our population health Gray Matter is thus firmly planted within the Sustainable Development Goals. There is nothing disruptive about it; it is simply a sustainable innovation (Christensen et al., 2015).

But why should governments around the world - nay - you the reader - care? It is an undeniable fact that migrant workers are trooping to the developed parts of the world to work as carers. Meanwhile as these migrants move from their home countries, oftentimes without the requisite documentation, they leave behind an already broken health system in the Low and Middle Income Countries.

The phenomenon of migrant workers sojourning in the advanced economies is a vicious cycle of rural-urban migration on a global scale. It will not stop until there is a concerted global effort and solidarity aimed at balancing the situation. You, as an individual, can do something about your home, your community, your village and your town/city. If you are an oldie reading this, you can express solidarity with your fellow senior citizens in other parts of the world who cannot afford a nursing care home or assisted living services.

You will notice that those with poorer healthcare systems also have a relatively smaller population of senior/ elderly people who are 60 years or older. This is because their older persons pop off from the population pyramid once they reach about age 60. That golden age, the age of retirement in many jurisdictions, is when they will need all the help they can get to take care of their health needs. You will also notice that those with better healthcare systems have the proportion of older persons aged 60 and above staying on top of the population pyramid well beyond age 60 into their 70s and 80s. The population pyramid graphs are sourced from www.populationpyramid.net and Jeff Desjardins/Visual Capitalist. This is done with a minimum narrative so that you may enter into your own interpretative understanding and draw your own additional conclusions. After you have studied the maps below, you may want to raise a debate about the relationship between income levels and the quality of care given to the aged.

Figure 1: A comparison of the 2017 population pyramids of the United States and
Nigeria

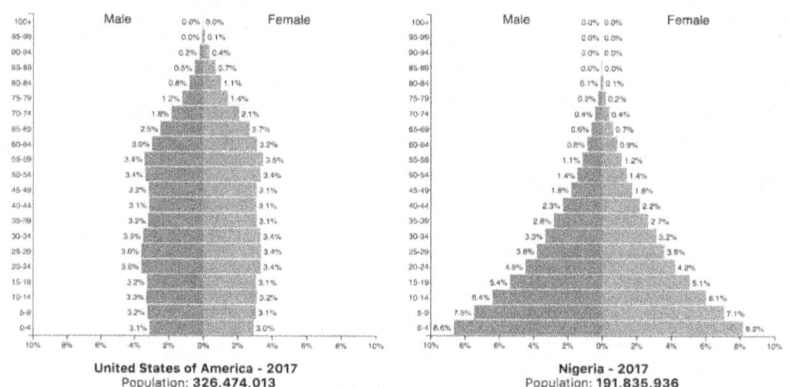

Source: Jeff Desjardins/Visual Capitalist; 2017 (Please see reference list for the link
to the website).

Nigeria is a Low and Middle Income Country and has a similar population growth
pattern as the Democratic Republic of Congo, and Ghana. Notice how Nigeria is
unable to keep its seniors by retirement age.

Figure 2: A comparison of Rapid, slow and negative population growth countries

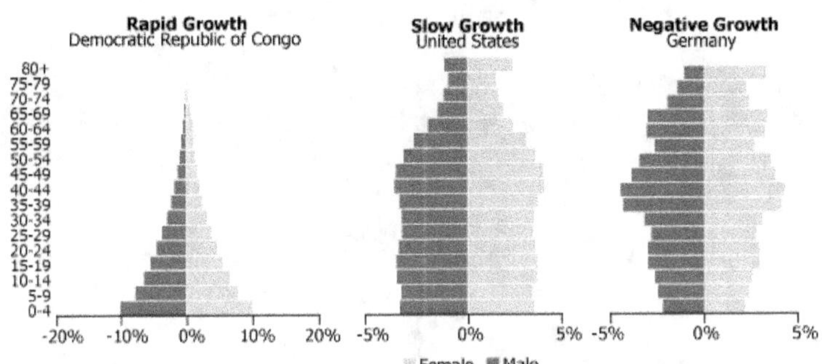

Source: Jeff Desjardins/Visual Capitalist; 2017 (Please see reference list for the link to the website).

Germany and the United States are of course developed countries with a similar population growth pattern, though Germany has a universal health insurance system. Did you notice the proportion of people aged 60 to 79 in Germany? How does that compare to that of the DRC?

Figure 3: Population pyramid of best practice Finland

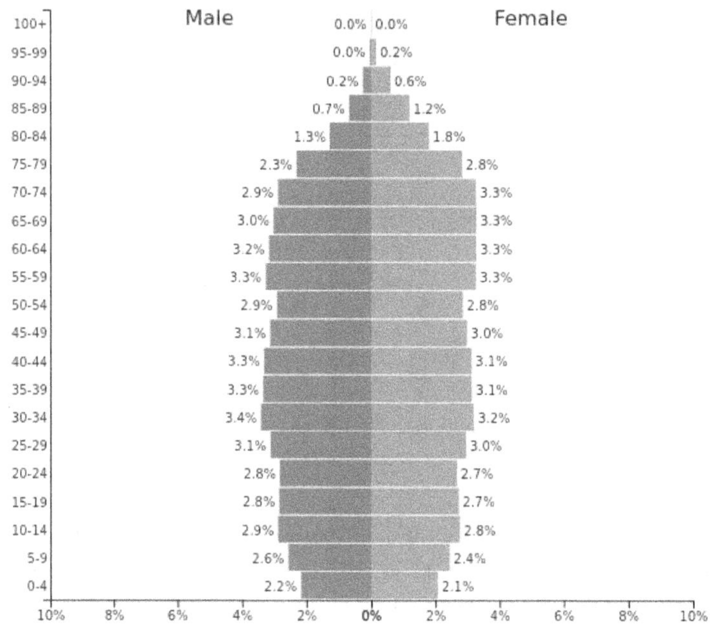

Figure 4: Population pyramid of Sweden - a model country for caregiving to the aged

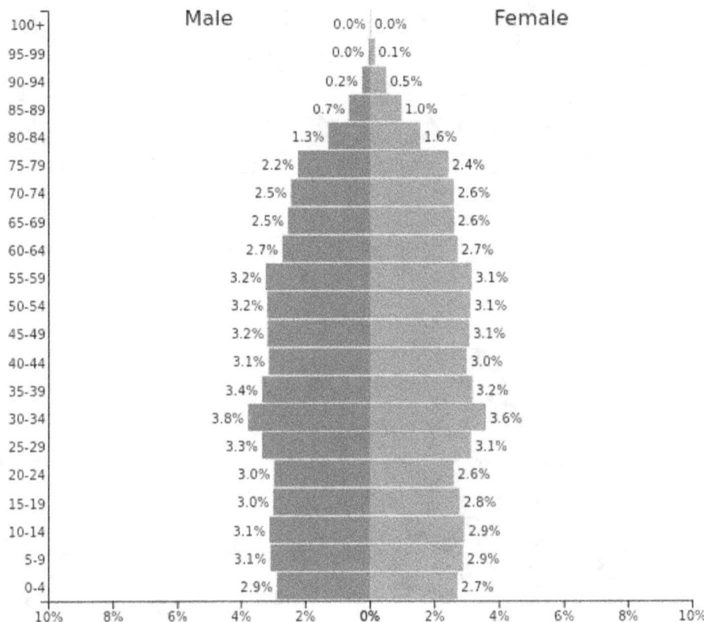

Figure 5: The 2020 Population pyramid of Ghana

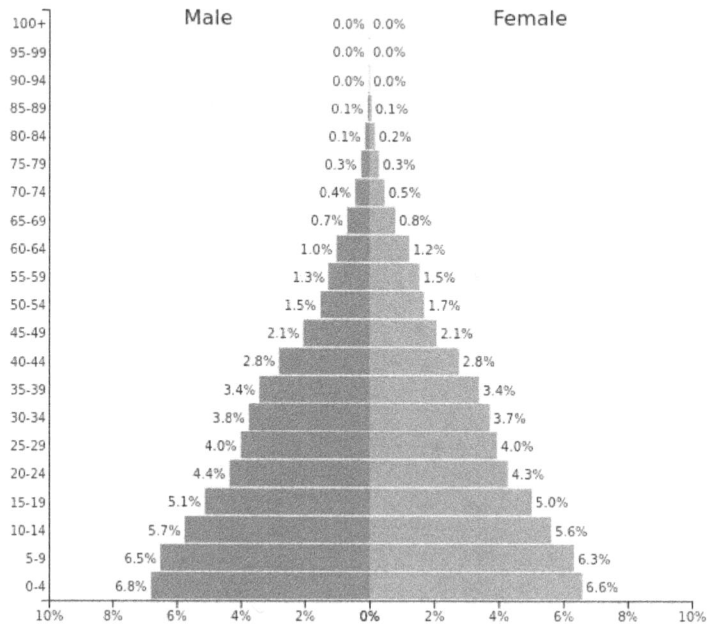

Male
Female
0.0% 0.0%
0.0% 0.0%
0.0% 0.0%
0.1% 0.1%
0.1% 0.2%
0.3% 0.3%
0.4% 0.5%
0.7% 0.8%
1.0% 1.2%
1.3% 1.5%
1.5% 1.7%
2.1% 2.1%
2.8% 2.8%
3.4% 3.4%
3.8% 3.7%
4.0% 4.0%
4.4% 4.3%
5.1% 5.0%
5.7% 5.6%
6.5% 6.3%
6.8% 6.6%
100+
95-99
90-94
85-89
80-84
75-79
70-74
65-69
60-64
55-59
50-54
45-49
40-44
35-39
30-34
25-29
20-24
15-19
10-14
5-9
0-4
10% 8% 6% 4% 2% 0% 2% 4% 6% 8% 10%
PopulationPyramid.net
Ghana - 2020
Population: 32,180,401

Figure 6: The 2050 population pyramid of Ghana

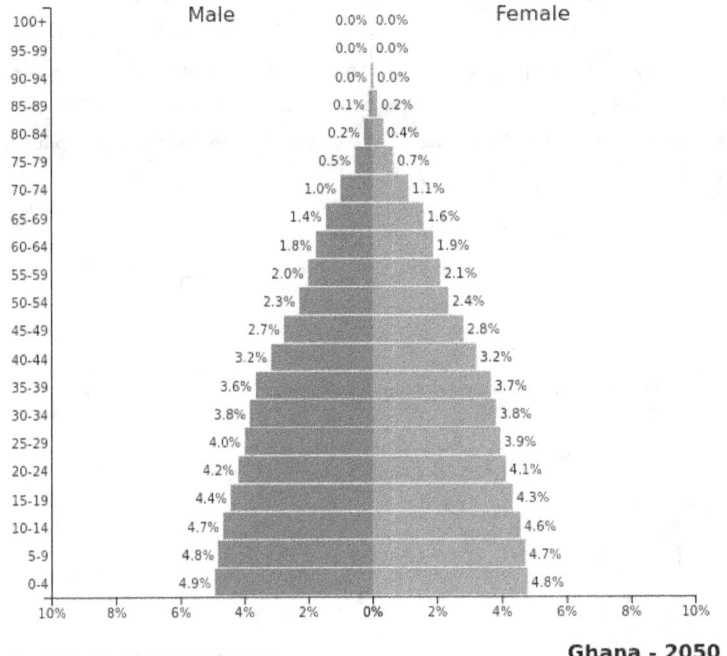

Please look carefully at figures 5 and 6, and compare them to the population pyramid of Nigeria in Figure 1 and the DRC in Figure 2. Do you foresee/agree that by 2050 the plight of seniors in those countries and in Low and Middle Income Countries generally will be the same if there is no population health intervention?

Now let's turn our attention to the Russian Federation (Figure 7), Canada (Figure 8) and China (Figure 9). Do they have a similar population structure for persons aged 60 and above? If you live in any of these three countries, what is your experience of home or nursing care home caregiving for the aged? Do you foresee illegal immigrants surviving your system? If you do not live in any of these countries, but have a relative living there, how do you foresee their plight in old age, a period of vulnerability?

Figure 7: Population pyramid of Russian Federation

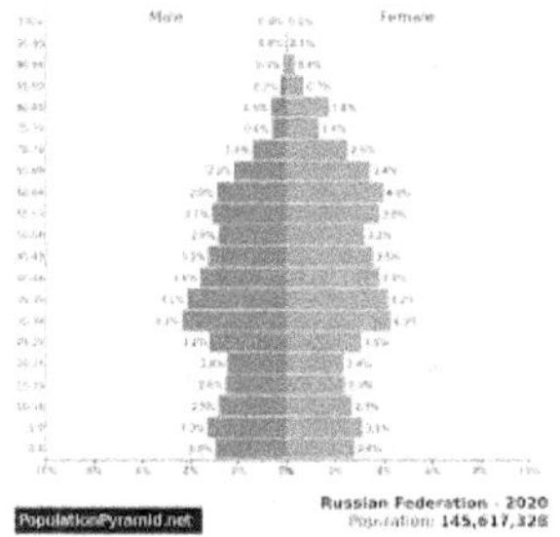

Figure 8: Population pyramid of Canada

In Russia universal healthcare coverage is enshrined in the Constitution under the Program of State Guarantees for Medical Care (PSG) (Somanathan et al., 2018). "The prevention and the early detection of diseases have developed intensively" in Russia today (Shishkin et al., 2022, para. 3).

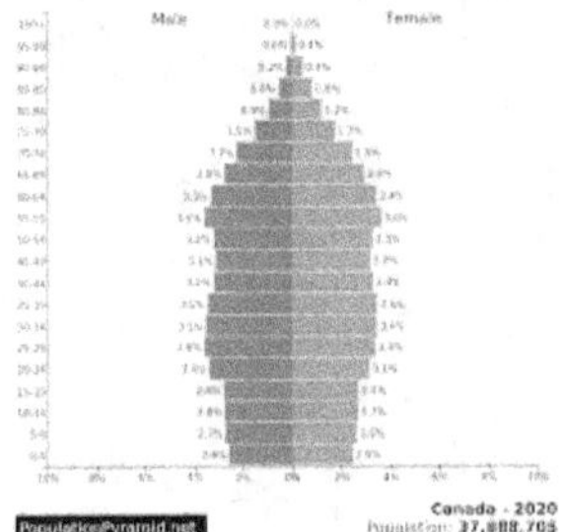

Figure 9: Population pyramid of China

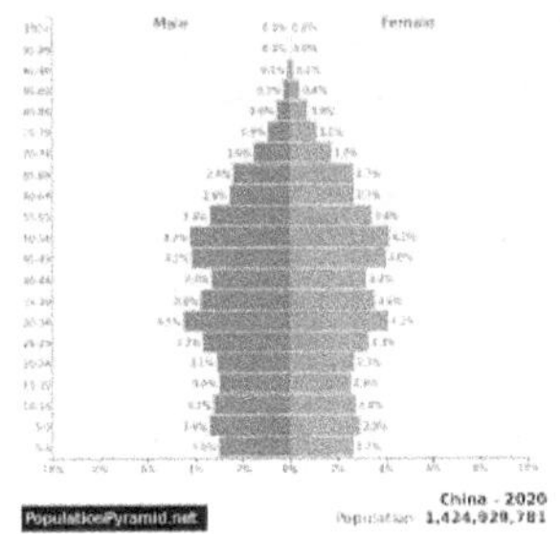

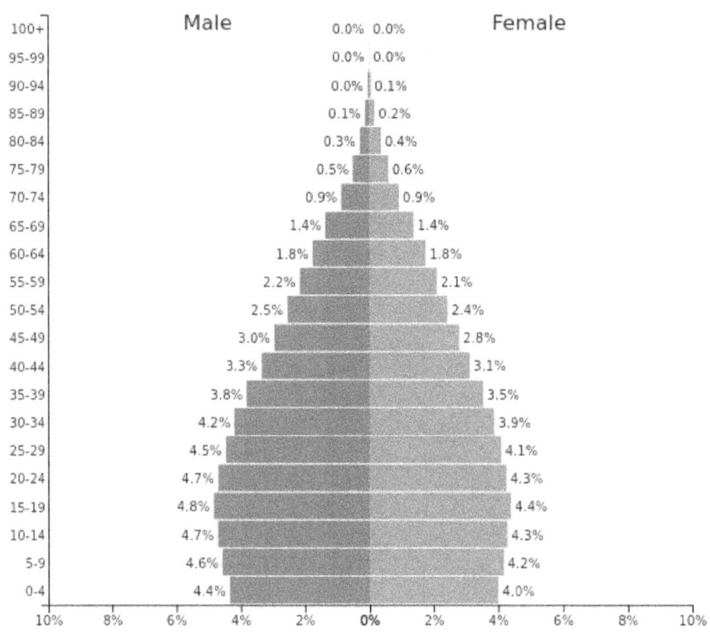

According to Wasserman (2022), Italy, South Korea, and Puerto Rico have a top heavy population pyramid with low fertility rates of less than 1.5 which has its own implications for assisted living and nursing care home services. "The population of older residents is also expanding, as life expectancy rises. In 2021, there were over 40 countries whose senior population (65+) was larger than its population of children (<15) and that number is expected to rise in the coming decades" (Wasserman, 2022, para. 4).

CONCLUSION

As Samuel Johnson rightly wrote on 10 November 1750 in The Rambler: "To be happy at home is the ultimate result of all ambition" (Taylor, 2018, para. 2). The framers of the U.S. constitution also famously declared, among other things, that all human beings are created equal, that they have inalienable rights; that among these are the right to life, liberty and the pursuit of happiness. Clearly, all human beings have the right to pursue happiness. We must hence all pursue safeguarding for the aged as a population health imperative. Our aged persons need to enjoy their last days, for, this is the desire of every human being.

If we die joyous, we're already in heaven. The time for global action and solidarity is now!

REFERENCES

Akdeniz, M., Yardımcı, B., & Kavukcu, E. (2021). Ethical considerations at the end-of-life care. *SAGE Open Medicine, 9*, 20503121211000918.

Acker, M., & Janssen, E. (2017). Are falls in the elderly less common in nursing homes compared with living at home?. *Evidence-Based Practice, 20*(2), 7-8. doi: 10.1097/01.EBP.0000541628.85587.81

alchemicalmedia. (2013, November 4). *Unseen tears: The native American boarding school experience in western New York part 1*[Video]. Youtube. https://www.youtube.com/watch?v=ioAzggmes8c

Agency for Healthcare Research and Quality. (2020, December). *2019 National healthcare quality and disparities report* (Pub. No. 20(21)-0045-EF). U.S. Department of Health and Human Services. https://www.ahrq.gov/research/findings/nhqrdr/nhqdr19/index.html

Alvarez, K.J., Kirchner, S., Chu, S., Smith, S., Winnick-Baskin, W., & Mielenz, T.J. (2015). Falls reduction and exercise training in an assisted living population. NCBI. https://www.ncbi.nlm.nih.gov/pmc/articles/PMC4541005/

American Association of Retired Persons. (2020, May). Age-friendly Seattle and King county, Washington, respond to COVID-19. AARP. https://www.aarp.org/livable-communities/network-age-friendly-communities/info-2020/seattle-king-county-washington-COVID-19-response.html

American Hospital Association, Committee on Research. (2014, January). *Your hospital's path to the second curve: Integration and transformation.* Health Research & Educational Trust. https://wgu.yourlearningportal.com/wgu/resources/courses/wgu_courses/hcm/mhl_v3/C990v3_MHL6610_integrated_health/resources/your_hospitals_path_second_curve.pdf

Anekar, A.A., Hendrix, J.M., & Cascella M. (2023). WHO analgesic ladder. In: StatPearls [Internet]. Treasure Island (FL): StatPearls Publishing. https://www.ncbi.nlm.nih.gov/books/NBK554435/

Badana, A.N.S., & Ross Andel, R. (2018). Aging in the Philippines. *The Gerontologist, 58*(2), 212–218. https://doi.org/10.1093/geront/gnx203

Bali, A.S., Howlett, M., Lewis, J.M., & Ramesh, M. (2021). Procedural policy tools in theory and practice, *Policy and Society, 40*(3), 295-311. DOI: 10.1080/14494035.2021.1965379

Becker's Hospital Review. (n.d.). 4 ways to ensure a successful hospital merger or acquisition. https://www.beckershospitalreview.com/hospital-transactions-and-valuation/4-ways-to-ensure-a-successful-hospital-merger-or-acquisition.html

BMA. (2017, March). Chronic pain: supporting safer prescribing of analgesics. https://www.bma.org.uk/media/2100/analgesics-chronic-pain.pdf

Boland, L., Légaré, F., Perez, M.M.B., Menear, M., Garvelink, M.M., McIsaac, D.I., Guérard, G.P., Emond, J., Brière, N., & Stacey, D. (2017, January 14). Impact of home care versus alternative locations of care on elder health outcomes: An overview of systematic reviews. *BMC Geriatrics, 17*(20). https://doi.org/10.1186/s12877-016-0395-y

Bu, F., Abell, J., Zaninotto, P., & Fancourt, D. (2020). A longitudinal analysis of loneliness, social isolation and falls amongst older people in England. *Scientific Reports, 10*(20064). https://doi.org/10.1038/s41598-020-77104-z

Burger, J. M. (2014). Situational features in Milgram's experiment that kept his participants shocking, *Journal of Social Issues, 70*(3), 489-500.

Category Archives: Ambiguous Images. (2018, August 20). A funny turn. https://www.opticalillusion.net/category/ambiguous-images/

Cao, H., & Chen, Z. (2018). The driving effect of internal and external environment on green innovation strategy-The moderating role of top management's environmental awareness. *Nankai Business Review International, 10*(3), 342-361.

Centers for Disease Control and Prevention. (n.d.). Prevent type 2 diabetes. https://www.cdc.gov/diabetes/prevent-type-2/index.html

Chinle Chapter Government. (2020). Welcome to the Chinle community. https://chinle.navajochapters.org/Default.aspx

Coe, C. (2021, April 5). Long-term care for the aged in Ghana is on the back burner. Here is how to change it. The Conversation. https://theconversation.com/long-term-care-for-the-aged-in-ghana-is-on-the-back-burner-here-is-how-to-change-it-158162

Christensen, C.M., Michael E. Raynor, M.E. & Rory McDonald, R. (2015, December). What Is disruptive innovation?. Harvard Business Review. https://www.google.com/amp/s/hbr.org/amp/2015/12/what-is-disruptive-innovation

County Health Rankings and Roadmap. (n.d.). King (KG). https://www.countyhealthrankings.org/app/washington/2021/rankings/king/county/outcomes/overall/snapshot

Cultural Learning Alliance. (2019, July 1). What is cultural capital? https://www.culturallearningalliance.org.uk/what-is-cultural-capital/#:~:text=Bourdieu%20believed%20that%20cultural%20capital,might%20call%20'high%20culture'.

Desjardins, J. (2017, September 28). Animation: Population pyramids of the 10 largest countries. Visual Capitalist. https://www.visualcapitalist.com/animation-population-pyramids-10-biggest-countries/

Devaney, M. (n.d.). Address these 3 critical risks before you start an assisted living home. Bplans.

https://articles.bplans.com/address-these-3-critical-risks-before-you-start-an-a
ssisted-living-home/

Dine College. (2019). Meet our faculty.
https://www.dinecollege.edu/academics/meet-our-faculty/

Durham, M. & Webb, S.S.N. (2014, October). Historical trauma: A panoramic
perspective. *The Brown University Child and Adolescent Behaviour
Newsletter, 30*(10).

Deneys-Tunney, A. (2012, July 15). Rousseau shows us that there is a way to break
the chains – from within. The Guardian.
https://www.theguardian.com/commentisfree/2012/jul/15/rousseau-shows-us-
way-break-chains

Emotion & Feeling. (n.d.). The Junto institute for entrepreneurial leadership.
https://www.thejuntoinstitute.com/emotion-wheels/

Felman, A. (2023, January 11). What is pain, and how do you treat it?. Medical
News Today. https://www.medicalnewstoday.com/articles/145750

Francis, G. (2005, January). Origins of the age 60 rule: A murky tale of power,
politics, and influence. Airline Pilot.
http://www3.alpa.org/portals/alpa/magazine/2005/Jan2005_originsage60rule.
htm

Gallanosa, A., Stevens, J.B.,& Quick, J. (2023). Glycopyrrolate. In: StatPearls
[Internet]. Treasure Island (FL): StatPearls
Publishing.https://www.ncbi.nlm.nih.gov/books/NBK526035/

Ghana Statistical Service. (2021, November). Ghana 2021 population and housing
census: General report volume 3A.
https://statsghana.gov.gh/gssmain/fileUpload/pressrelease/2021%20PHC%20
General%20Report%20Vol%203A_Population%20of%20Regions%20and%20D
istricts_181121.pdf

Giannulli, T. (2014, October 17). Four reasons to use online medical appointment
scheduling. *Physicians Practice, 24.*
https://www.physicianspractice.com/technology/four-reasons-use-online-medic
al-appointment-scheduling

Gladwell, M. (2008). *Outliers: The story of success.* Little, Brown and Company.

Hansen, A. (2021, September 15). Six forms of cultural wealth you can leverage as a
leader. The Glasshammer.
https://theglasshammer.com/2021/09/six-forms-of-cultural-wealth-you-can-lev
erage-as-a-leader/

Harris, N.B. (2014, September). *How childhood trauma affects health across a
lifetime* (Video). TED Conferences.
https://www.ted.com/talks/nadine_burke_harris_how_childhood_trauma_affec
ts_health_across_a_lifetime?language=en

Harvard University. (n.d.). ACEs and toxic stress: Frequently asked questions.
https://developingchild.harvard.edu/resources/aces-and-toxic-stress-frequentl
y-asked-questions/

Hardman, R.J., Kennedy, G., Macpherson, H., Scholey, A.B., & Pipingas, A. (2015). A randomised controlled trial investigating the effects of Mediterranean diet and aerobic exercise on cognition in cognitively healthy older people living independently within aged care facilities: The Lifestyle Intervention in Independent Living Aged Care (LIILAC) study protocol [ACTRN12614001133628]. *Nutrition Journal, 14*, 1-10. DOI: 10.1186/s12937-015-0042-z.

Haslam, S. A., Reicher, S.D., & Millard, K. (2015). Shock treatment: Using immersive digital realism to restage and re-examine Milgram's 'obedience to authority' research, *PLoS ONE, 10*(3), 1-10. https://doi.org/10.1371/journal.pone.0109015

Haslam, S.A. & Reicher, S.D. (2018). A truth that does not always speak its name: How Hollander and Turowetz's findings confirm and extend the engaged followership analysis of harm-doing in the Milgram paradigm, *British Journal of Social Psychology, 57*(2), 292-300.

Hatcher, T.L. (2020, October 16). Elderly fall prevention in assisted living facilities. Relias. https://www.relias.com/blog/reducing-preventing-falls-elderly-adults

Healy, P. (2017, June 8). The fundamental attribution error: What it is & how to avoid it. Harvard Business School Online. https://online.hbs.edu/blog/post/the-fundamental-attribution-error

Health Research and Educational Trust. (2013, April). Metrics for the second curve of health care. http://www.hpoe.org/Reports-HPOE/Metrics_Second_Curve_4_13.pdf

Heath, S. (2018, January 3). Exploring open access scheduling in patient access to care. Patient Engagement Hit. https://patientengagementhit.com/news/exploring-open-access-scheduling-in-patient-access-to-care

Ilunga, P. (2022, June 5). Belgian King admits colonial wrongs, but declines to apologise. The East African. https://www.theeastafrican.co.ke/tea/rest-of-africa/belgian-king-colonial-wrongs-congo-3843580

Jahromi, V. K., Tabatabaee, S. S., Abdar, Z. E., & Rajabi, M. (2016). Active listening: The key of successful communication in hospital managers. *Electronic Physician, 8*(3), 2123–2128. https://doi.org/10.19082/2123

Johnson, C. (2022, July 28). How to be happy according to Plato. The Collector. https://www.thecollector.com/how-to-be-happy-according-to-plato/

Jouffre, S., & Croizet, J-C. (2016). Empowering and legitimizing the fundamental attribution error: Power and legitimization exacerbate the translation of role-constrained behaviors into ability differences, *European Journal of Social Psychology, 46*(5), 621-631. https://doi.org/10.1002/ejsp.2191

Ketcham, C., & Knight, K.W. (2014). Strategy, constraint, risk management and the value chain. In J-P Louisot, & C.H. Ketcham (Eds.), *ERM - Enterprise risk management issues and cases* (pp. 12-19), John Wiley & Sons, Incorporated.

Khimm, S. (2021, March 7). America now knows that nursing homes are broken. Does anyone care enough to fix them?. NBC Universal. https://www.nbcnews.com/politics/politics-news/america-now-knows-nursing-homes-are-broken-does-anyone-care-n1259766

Klimova, B., Maresova, P., Valis, M., Hort, J., & Kuca, K. (2015). Alzheimer's disease and language impairments: social intervention and medical treatment. *Clinical Interventions in Aging, 10*, 1401–1407. https://doi.org/10.2147/CIA.S89714

Kingcountyemployees. (2021, October 7). Indigenous peoples' day to be an observed holiday beginning in 2022. King County. https://kcemployees.com/2021/10/07/indigenous-peoples-day-to-be-an-observed-holiday-beginning-in-2022/

King County. (n.d.). Long-term care facility data dashboard. https://kingcounty.gov/depts/health/covid-19/data/LTCF.aspx

Knight Lozano, R., May, S., Clarkson, C., & Sarjeant, R. (2021). Caregiver experiences of paediatric inpatient cardiac services: A qualitative systematic review. *European Journal of Cardiovascular Nursing, 20*(2), 147–159. https://doi.org/10.1177/1474515120951974

Kovacevic, D. (2022, August 18). The 20 richest countries in the world right now might surprise you. https://www.slice.ca/the-20-richest-countries-in-the-world-right-now-might-surprise-you/

Kyei-Baafour, E., Tornyigah, B., Buade, B., Bimi, L., Oduro, A. R., Koram, K. A., Gyan, B. A., & Kusi, K. A. (2020). Impact of an irrigation dam on the transmission and diversity of *Plasmodium falciparum* in a seasonal malaria transmission area of northern Ghana. *Journal of Tropical Medicine*, 1386587. https://doi.org/10.1155/2020/1386587

Kwanzaa, B.K. (2020, November 12). Understanding the intra-ethnic conflict in Bimbilla. Danish Institute for International Studies. https://www.diis.dk/en/node/24350#:~:text=The%20northern%20parts%20of%20Ghana,on%20the%20other%2C%20among%20others.

Lai, C. (2022). More than carrots and sticks: Economic statecraft and coercion in China–Taiwan relations from 2000 to 2019. *Politics, 42*(3), 410-425.

Lally, M. & Valentine-French, S. (2020, December 6). Heredity, prenatal development, and birth. Social Science.

Lighter, D. (2011). Basics of health care performance improvement. Western Governors University. https://wgu.vitalsource.com/#/books/9781284061260/cfi/6/2!/4/2@0:0

Leath, B.A., Dunn, L.W. Alsobrook, A., & Darden, M.L. (2018). Enhancing rural population health care access and outcomes through the telehealth

EcoSystem™ model. *Online Journal Public Health Informatics, 10*(2), e218. doi: 10.5210/ojphi.v10i2.9311

Lee, L.W., & Fiore, R.A. (2020). Measuring levels of fundamental attribution error ascribed to leadership of entrepreneurial organizations across national cultures, *Journal of Business Strategies, 37*(1), 1-28.

Liu, Z., Heffernan, C., & Tan, J. (2020). Caregiver burden: A concept analysis. *International journal of nursing sciences, 7*(4), 438–445. https://doi.org/10.1016/j.ijnss.2020.07.012

Mayo Clinic. (n.d.). Midazolam (injection route). https://www.mayoclinic.org/drugs-supplements/midazolam-injection-route/description/drg-20064813

McCoy, C. A. (2019). Adapting coercion: how three industrialized nations manufacture vaccination compliance. *Journal of Health Politics, Policy and Law, 44*(6), 823-854.

McLeod, S. (2017). The Milgram shock experiment. Simply Psychology. https://www.simplypsychology.org/milgram.html

McPherson, M.B.; & Young, S.L. (2004). What students think when teachers get upset: fundamental attribution error and student-generated reasons for teacher anger. *Communication Quarterly, 52*(4), 357-369. https://doi.org/10.1080/01463370409370206

Mensah, I.A. (2023). *Poems and their meanings.* Amazon. https://www.amazon.com/POEMS-THEIR-MEANINGS-Isaac-Mensah-ebook/dp/B0C6NZLG8B/ref=sr_1_2?qid=1686911158&refinements=p_27%3AIsaac+Ato++Mensah&s=digital-text&sr=1-2&text=Isaac+Ato++Mensah

Mensah, I.A.. (2020, August 17). The mudslinging must cease now: A short primer on ethics and personality attacks. Writers & Shakespeares Ghana Limited. https://www.writersghana.com/index.php/2020/08/17/the-mudslinging-must-cease-now-a-short-primer-on-ethics-and-personality-attacks/

Mensah, I.A. (2019a). Why IYIL2019 is important for Ghana. Writers & Shakespeares Ghana Limited. https://www.writersghana.com/index.php/2019/01/07/why-iyil2019-is-important-for-ghana/

Mensah, I.A. (2019b). All souls day, ghosts and our demons. Writers & Shakespeares Ghana Limited. https://www.writersghana.com/index.php/2019/11/07/all-souls-day-ghosts-and-our-demons/

Mensah, I.A. (2018, September 29). Were you forced to sign the ECOWAS protocol? The million dollar question on alphabetical literacy. Writers & Shakespeares Ghana Limited. https://www.writersghana.com/index.php/2018/09/29/were-you-forced-to-sign-the-ecowas-protocol-the-million-dollar-question-on-alphabetical-literacy/

Miller, C. (n.d.). Impact assessment framework. Western Governors University. https://wgu.yourlearningportal.com/wgu/resources/courses/wgu_courses/hcm/

mhl/C984_MHL5510_financial_management/resources/impact_assessment_fr
amework.pdf

Moran, J.M., Jolly, E., & Mitchell, J.P. (2014). Spontaneous mentalizing predicts the fundamental attribution error. *Journal of Cognitive Neuroscience, 26*(3), 569-576. https://doi.org/10.1162/jocn_a_00513

NACHC. (2014, October 22). *What is a community health center?* [Video]. Youtube. https://www.youtube.com/watch?v=NSGIrdNnRvw

National Ageing Policy: 'Ageing with Security and Dignity'. (2010). Ministry of Gender, Children and Social Protection. https://www.mogcsp.gov.gh/mdocs-posts/national-ageing-policy-ageing-with-se curity-and-dignity/

National Geographic. (2015, November 4). *Is that my real hand? Breakthrough* [Video]. Youtube. https://www.youtube.com/watch?v=DphlhmtGRqI

National Institute for Health and Care Excellence. (n.d.). Advance care planning. https://www.nice.org.uk/about/nice-communities/social-care/quick-guides/adva nce-care-planning

Nimo, K.K. (2022, August 24). Bold style reigned supreme at Ghana's Chale Wote festival. Vogue. https://www.vogue.com/slideshow/chale-wote-street-style-2022

North African Post. (2016, January 23). Côte d'Ivoire-Morocco: 100 Ivorian preachers to be trained in Mohammed VI Institute. https://northafricapost.com/10616-cote-divoire-morocco-100-ivorian-preachers -to-be-trained-in-mohammed-vi-institute.html

Neufeld, J. (2017, January 14). Nursing home and long term care demographics. Elder Needs Law. https://www.elderneedslaw.com/blog/how-many-older-adults-will-wind-up-in-s killed-nursing-homes#:~:text=In%202030%2C%20almost%2070%20million,in %20time%20in%20their%20lives.

OECD. (2015). *Health at a glance 2015: OECD indicators.* OECD Publishing. https://doi.org/10.1787/health_glance-2015-en.

Ohio University. (n.d.). The ADDRESSING model. https://www.ohio.edu/cas/psychology/diversity/addressing-model

Oswalt, A. (n.d.). Urie Bronfenbrenner and child development. Southeastern Arizona Behavioral Health Services, Inc. https://www.seabhs.org/poc/view_doc.php?type=doc&id=7930&cn=28

Roser, M., Ortiz-Ospina, E., & Ritchie, H. (2019, October). Life expectancy. Our World in Data. https://ourworldindata.org/life-expectancy#:~:text=No%20country%20in%20t he%20world,is%20now%20above%2070%20years.

Rural Health Information Hub. (n.d.). Demographic changes and aging population. https://www.ruralhealthinfo.org/toolkits/aging/1/demographics#:~:text=Today %2C%20there%20are%20more%20than,increase%20by%20almost%2018%20 million

Russell, R.J. (n.d.). John Paul II on science and religion: A deeply appreciative
    reflection. Interdisciplinary Encyclopedia of Religion and Science.
    https://inters.org/reflection-on-John-Paul-II-science-religion
Sangeetha, T., Kumutha, D., Divya Bharathi, M., & Surendran, R. (2022). Smart
    mattress integrated with pressure sensor and IoT functions for sleep apnea
    detection. *Measurement: Sensors, 24*(100450).
    https://doi.org/10.1016/j.measen.2022.100450.
Schulz, R., & Sherwood, P. R. (2008). Physical and mental health effects of family
    caregiving. *The American Journal of Nursing, 108*(9 Suppl), 23–27.
    https://doi.org/10.1097/01.NAJ.0000336406.45248.4c
Sharma, S. (2023, April 10). Ambulance crisis 'horror' forcing Britons to make their
    own way to hospital. Independent.
    https://www.independent.co.uk/news/health/ambulance-delays-nhs-crisis-east
    er-strike-b2317000.html
Shishkin, S., Sheiman, I., Vlassov, V., Potapchik, E., & Sazhina, S. (2022).
    Structural changes in the Russian health care system: Do they match
    European trends?. *Health Econ Rev,* 12(29).
    https://doi.org/10.1186/s13561-022-00373-z
Somanathan, A., Sheiman, I., Salakhutdinova, S., & Buisman, L. (2018, August 15).
    Universal health coverage in Russia: Extending coverage for the poor in the
    post-Soviet era. The World Bank Group.
    https://elibrary.worldbank.org/doi/abs/10.1596/30026
St Christopher's. (n.d.). Quality of care.
    https://www.stchristophers.org.uk/quality-of-care
Substance Abuse and Mental Health Services Administration. (2009, January).
    CultureCard: A guide to build cultural awareness. U.S. Department of Health
    and Human Services.
    https://store.samhsa.gov/product/American-Indian-and-Alaska-Native-Cul
    ture-Card/sma08-4354
Taylor, T. (2018, December 26). To be happy at home is the ultimate result of all
    ambition. Conversable Economist.
    https://conversableeconomist.blogspot.com/2018/12/to-be-happy-at-home-is-ul
    timate-result.html
The Danish Institute for Human Rights. (n.d.). Goals, targets and indicators.
    https://sdg.humanrights.dk/en/goals-and-targets
The World Bank. (2022, August 22). The World Bank in middle income countries.
    https://www.worldbank.org/en/country/mic/overview
Then & Now. (2019, December 14). *Bourdieu: Cultural capital, the love of art & hip
    hop* [Video]. Youtube. https://www.youtube.com/watch?v=th0eYWnGZ_4
Turkheimer, E. (n.d.). The nature-nurture question.
    https://nobaproject.com/modules/the-nature-nurture-question

United States Census Bureau. (n.d.). QuickFacts King county, Washington.
    https://www.census.gov/quickfacts/kingcountywashington

Waldinger, R. (2015, November). *Robert Waldinger: What makes a good life? Lessons from the longest study on happiness* [Video]. TED Conferences. https://youtu.be/8KkKuTCFvzI

Wasserman, P. (2022, April 20).What is a negative, or top-heavy, population pyramid?. Population Education. https://populationeducation.org/what-is-a-negative-or-top-heavy-population-pyramid/

Waters, S. (2023, May 18). What's a vocation? 8 tips for finding yours. BetterUp. https://www.betterup.com/blog/what-is-a-vocation

World Health Organization. (n.d.). Ghana: Health data overview for the Republic of Ghana. https://data.who.int/countries/288

World Population Review. (n.d.). Happiest countries in the world 2023. https://worldpopulationreview.com/country-rankings/happiest-countries-in-the-world

United Nations. (n.d.). Conferences: Aging. https://www.un.org/en/conferences/ageing

University of Washington. (n.d.). What is population health?. https://www.washington.edu/populationhealth/about/what-is-population-health/

Yosso, T.J. (2005). Whose culture has capital? A critical race theory discussion of community cultural wealth. *Race Ethnicity and Education, 8*(1), 69-91. DOI: 10.1080/1361332052000341006

Zhao, P., Yoo, I., Lavoie, J., Lavoie, J. B., & Simoes, E. (2017, April 26). Web-based medical appointment systems: A systematic review. *NIH: National Library of Medicine. Med Internet Res, 19*(4), e134. doi: 10.2196/jmir.6747.

Safeguarding the aged is such an important concept - a gray matter. An entire life's career spent working in a nursing care home, or residential care home, may not be enough to guarantee an error-free, litigation-free caregiving. Besides, we all desire to grow old. Hence, we may at some period in our lives need help with assisted living. Therefore, this book is for you who need to refresh your mind about caring for your aged relatives - nay, about yourself, before it's too late! It draws on best practice experiences/practices from the US and UK, as well as the latest reference material on safeguarding. The authors share their real, practical experiences with you in order to show you the care given to your aged relatives in a nursing care home/ residential care home. Thereby, the book exposes you to the care you will receive as a senior. The authors advocate safeguarding the aged as a population health concept within the Sustainable Development Goals. We know for sure that you have empathy/sympathy for the elderly persons close to you. Yes, that's why you have grabbed this book, isn't it? It is written by healthcare practitioners who have had - and still have - direct engagement with residents/patients. The authors also offer perspectives on safeguarding from a Low and Middle Income Country - Ghana - thereby helping to decolonize the curriculum. Now you have the raison d'etre and know-how of caregiving, whether at home, a residential care home, or in a nursing care home. It will help you shape up for the inevitable gray matter that is staring you in the mirror now.

ABOUT THE AUTHORS

Isaac Ato Mensah is an independent scholar and journalist based in Accra, Ghana. He previously worked as a professionally trained Health Services Administrator for about 10 years at a non-profit Catholic Mission hospital, a government hospital, and a private for-profit hospital. He was also a lecturer at three private university colleges in Accra. He is a founding editorial board member of the Tema Medical Journal published by Narh-Bita College, Tema, Ghana. Isaac Ato Mensah holds a bachelor's degree in Health Services Administration from the School of Administration (now renamed University of Ghana Business School), University of Ghana, Legon, Accra. He also holds a master of arts degree in Communication Studies from the same university.

Florence Afful is a Registered General Nurse. She started her career in 1998 as a bedside Nurse at the Komfo Anokye Teaching Hospital (KATH) in Kumasi, Ghana. From there she continued her bedside nursing at Nkawie District Hospital, Kumasi. Later, she continued her bedside nursing at the Korle Bu Teaching Hospital in Accra, Ghana. She has since 2004 - that is, for at least 18 years - worked as a nurse at Albany Nursing Home in Croydon, London, a facility managed by the Future Care Group of the UK. Her concentrated effort and expertise has no doubt led to the recognition of the Future Care Group as one of the Top 20 recommended care home groups in the UK by carehome.co.uk, one of the UK's leading care home review websites. Florence Afful (formerly known as Florence Afful) completed her State Registered Nurse training at Komfo Anokye Nurses Training College (NTC), Kumasi in Ghana, now renamed Nursing and Midwifery Training College, Kumasi.

Edem Yao Ahiati worked as a Senior Assistance Center Manager at the National Asian Pacific Center on Aging, Seattle, Washington, USA. Before moving to the state of Washington, he played a similar role in Albany, NY. His daily routine involved assisting clients with accessing their claims on Medicare, Medicaid, Affordable Care Act, Essential Plan, Qualified Health Plan, Health Plan Benefits, Eligibility, Claims, Complaints and Appeals, Precertification, Referrals, Diagnosis Codes, etc. Most of his direct client engagement involved assisting thousands of elderly people one-on-one over the telephone and via email to access their health insurance claims. Edem Ahiati holds a master of Health Leadership degree from Western Governors University, USA.

Barbara Vanessa Sabbi is a Certified Nursing Assistant (CNA). She has worked at Weatherly Inn, Tacoma, Washington, USA since 2019. Her work includes bathing and grooming patients with low mobility; helping them follow their diet plan, take in their medications and walk; and monitoring their behavior. A significant number of the residents she gives care to are persons living with dementia, Alzheimer's Disease and other comorbidities.

Barbara Sabbi is a student at Tacoma Community College, Washington State, USA.